W9-BMY-822

BEAT DIABETES!

How I Overcame Diabetes and You Can Too!

MARGARET BLACKSTONE

Adams Media Corporation
Holbrook, Massachusetts

Copyright ©2000, Margaret Blackstone. All rights reserved.
This book, or parts thereof, may not be reproduced in any
form without permission from the publisher; exceptions are made for
brief excerpts used in published reviews.

Published by
Adams Media Corporation
260 Center Street, Holbrook, MA 02343

ISBN: 1-58062-183-X

Printed in the United States of America.

J I H G F E D C B A

Library of Congress Cataloging-in-Publication Data
Blackstone, Margaret.
Beat diabetes! : how I overcame diabetes and you can too! /
Margaret Blackstone.
        p.   cm.
ISBN 1-58062-183-X
1. Non-insulin-dependent diabetes—Treatment. 2. Low-carbohydrate diet. I. Title.
    RC662.18.B585   1999
    616.4'6206—dc21   99-15823
                CIP

Many of the designations used by manufactures and sellers to distinguish their products are claimed as trademarks. Where those designations have appear in this book
and Adams Media was aware of a trademark claim, the designations have been printed
in initial capital letters.

This publication is designed to provide accurate and authoritative information with
regard to the subject matter covered. It is sold with the understanding that the publisher
is not engaged in rendering professional medical advice. If assistance is required, the
services of a competent professional person should be sought.

This book is available at quantity discounts for bulk purchases.
For information, call 1-800-872-5627.

Visit our home page at http://www.adamsmedia.com

This book is dedicated with love to Channa Taub
and Carol Mann, and they know all the
many reasons why.

Acknowledgments

Thank you to my son Dash Lunde, my mother Barbara Blackstone, dear friend and fine wordsmith, Trent Duffy, Clover Laleazhar, Pam Liflander, Sarah Larson, Marie Maes, and my doctors, Marty Beitler, MD, Richard Bernstein, MD, and my meditative endocrinoligist, Andrew Jay Drexler, M.D., who helps make balance a way of life. Thanks.

Let me also acknowledge three friends whose lives might have been saved had we known then what we know now: Walter Clemons, Joe Schaeffer, and Milton Sherman.

Contents

PART 1
Welcome to My Pancreas

PART 2
Tight Control Keeps the Doctor Away

PART 3
Prevention, Permanent

PART 4
The Art of the Diet

PART 5
The Sisyphus Strategy:
Lift Weights, Walk Uphill, Don't Stop

PART 6
Methodology Over Matter:
Contributions to a Centered Life

Introduction

When making a wish list, no one puts being diagnosed with diabetes at the top. So I'm not going to be the Pollyanna of the blood glucose set and say that diabetes is the greatest thing that ever happened to me; chances are it won't be the greatest thing since sliced bread for you either. (That's okay, because bread is one of the foods we healthy diabetics need to avoid. It's too high in carbohydrates, which raise blood glucose levels in the first place and unduly tax whatever insulin your pancreas may still be producing.)

But how you deal with diabetes will teach you a lot about yourself, and managing diabetes well can and will change your life for the better, as long as you are willing to accept the challenge. So please bear with me when I say that this is an exciting time to be a diabetic. Once the poor stepsister of serious diseases, diabetes is finally coming into its own. More dollars are being allotted for research, and the treatment of diabetes is undergoing a sorely needed overhaul. Instead of accepting that even with the aid of insulin injections or oral hypoglycemic agents, many diabetics will still have to live with elevated blood sugar, more and more informed diabetologists are concentrating on upholding the equal rights of all diabetics to reach and maintain normal blood glucose levels through individualized treatment protocols, thereby minimizing the risk of complications later in the disease—complications that can take the life of a diabetic when they become severe enough. When it comes to diabetes treatment, the tectonic plates of the Old Guard treatment are finally shifting.

Thank goodness, because until recently, diabetics have languished in a quagmire of inaccurate treatment and a disheartening outlook, and while the number of people suffering from some life-threatening diseases, like heart disease, is on the wane, the number of those who suffer from diabetes is on the rise. This is partly because ours is a sedentary culture; despite the popularity of diet and exercise programs, obesity (a major risk factor for diabetes in adults) is a problem for the majority of the population. In addition, people are living longer, and as with most diseases, the risk for diabetes increases with age. But there are two unique reasons that the number of diabetics is increasing: (1) diabetes is not yet on our "most wanted list" of diseases to cure, and (2) to this day, the disease is misunderstood and even mistreated by many doctors.

Unfortunately, we diabetics still get a bum rap. I saw this in the reactions of many people I told immediately following my diagnosis. "Oh, isn't that when you lose a limb?" "Gosh, does that mean you're going to lose your eyesight?" You'd think we were lepers or something. (Not that there is anything wrong with lepers. As a matter of fact, leprosy and diabetes share the burden of often being misunderstood by the general public.) Faced with such a negative image of the disease, many of us feel defeated, even depressed, when diagnosed. But, as I hope to show you, it's possible to feel challenged and inspired. Rather than thinking of diabetes as a disease, you may want to view it as a chronic condition, one that you can control, if you try. Instead of feeling you've lost the battle before you begin, tell yourself that you haven't even begun to fight.

One reason being diagnosed with diabetes comes as such a blow is that we tend to confuse diabetes with the complications that can occur when the condition isn't well managed. Giving the complications center stage before you even get started on coping with the diagnosis is akin to taking a first-time visitor to this country to Sing Sing, and saying, "Okay. Here you go. This is the United States." Any normal person would run in the opposite direction.

The same problem occurs with diabetes and its complications. The two are not synonymous. Complications occur only when blood glucose levels are haywire for a long period of time. In other words, if you can keep your blood glucose levels consistently in the normal range, you are as normal as the next person. You won't have complications; ergo you won't feel as if you have a disease. In fact, you may feel a little healthier than many of your non-diabetic friends, since you are taking such good care of yourself.

Similarly, how you view diabetes and how you respond to your own diagnosis will have a major impact on how healthy a life you can continue to have. If you regard diabetes as a deadly disease, the diagnosis can seem a defeat, and diabetes your antagonist. You may feel that this news threatens your way of life. With that attitude, the odds are high that you will not succeed in taking good care of yourself (the kind of care that will keep you symptom-free) and that you'll have to contend with the risk of complications. On the other hand, you can view diabetes as a condition, the diagnosis as an invisible presence that eggs you on to invest in caring for yourself more than ever. You'll then feel motivated to do a little bit better every day and to take advantage of this wake-up call to be healthier than you were before.

Without a doubt, probably the hardest thing for anyone to do in life is to take care of themselves. It's just a whole lot more complicated than most of us let on. Consider diabetes your invitation to do just that—take care of yourself—and you're on your way to a better life. When tender loving care is a must, you might just find you're capable of it, and I mean with yourself.

To hear from many people who have been diagnosed, you would think diabetes develops overnight. But this is not the case. As for those people who seemed to be diabetes-free one day and a diabetic the next, unfortunately most of them have been diabetic for some time—enough time for the diabetes to have already caused damage.

Diabetes is basically a condition of both internal accretion and attrition—*accretion* because as your blood glucose becomes consistently elevated, damage builds up and *attrition* because as your blood glucose levels begin to elevate, the insulin you do produce becomes less and less able to process the glucose in your system. In a process almost akin to friction, the power of the insulin you do produce wears away. This book is for diabetics and those who are at risk for diabetes. Those with a proclivity to develop diabetes include anyone who is at higher risk for diabetes than the general public. *Beat Diabetes!* can help you prevent the consequences of the disease, and if you don't "have" it yet but are at risk, it may even help you prevent the disease.

If all the confusion, misinformation, and misunderstanding that surround the definition and the diagnosis of diabetes were not enough, there is the added problem that the treatment itself can lead to the serious complications that it supposedly protects against. Drug treatment, coupled with the high-carbohydrate diet prescribed for diabetics, can leave the newly diagnosed diabetic not much better off than the diabetic who hasn't been diagnosed at all. As I'll describe in detail later, carbohydrate—the compound that insulin breaks down into fuel for the body—is what the doctor ordered, but it's just what the diabetic can't handle.

The prescribed insulin and oral agents are supposed to assist in this inadequate digestive process. It's analogous to the "coals to Newcastle syndrome"—coals (carbohydrates) are being hauled to Newcastle, and the fires (the drugs) must grow bigger and brighter simply to dispose of the additional, unwanted coals. Although the coals in the scenario may not be intrinsically harmful, carbohydrates can be. When the process doesn't work efficiently—as very often happens—many physicians go on to prescribe higher doses of oral medication or insulin. Life for the diabetic can only get worse as he or she continues to "feed the medication." The very treatment that is supposed to protect the diabetic can contribute to the serious complications of the disease over the long term.

Until recently, such a treatment plan was never even questioned, and certainly patients didn't question their doctors about health issues. Newly diagnosed patients are usually terrified by the bleak picture painted in medical texts and by physicians regarding the debilitating side effects that can occur in extreme, long-term cases of diabetes. Spurred on by the negative propaganda, they willingly acquiesce to do "whatever's necessary." The assumption passed on to the patient is that "aggressive" treatment (with drugs) will prevent complications.

In truth, keeping blood glucose levels consistently normal avoids further complications—however you get there. In fact, such side effects as gangrene and blindness occur only in situations in which blood glucose levels have been out of control for many years. (Sadly the overtreatment prescribed for diabetes can contribute to rapid and extreme fluctuations in those levels, and major and recurrent shifts in amplitude can be as damaging as chronically high blood sugar. The two together are ultimately poison.) Whereas when blood glucose levels are kept in tight control—in the normal range and without a great deal of variation—the risk of such complications is minimal to nonexistent. Yet this motivating factor is rarely part of the speech new diabetics receive from their physicians. Instead, what is very much in their control (their blood glucose levels) is presented as being out of their control.

Now, you can change all that with the help of this book. The regimen outlined here will still seem unorthodox to many doctors, even though the proof is in the result—normal blood sugar. The basic premise is to reverse the dietary emphasis, shifting the central component of your diet from carbohydrate to protein and, because anaerobic exercise burns glucose, making anaerobic exercise a major part of your exercise regimen.

Most other books on diabetes still recommend the opposite approach—a high carbohydrate diet and plenty of aerobic exercise. Many reputable medical institutions also advocate this "Old Guard" diabetes treatment, as does the American Diabetes Association. What does this mean? Simply that all of these programs are behind the curve when it comes to diabetes research and treatment and that patients following these regimens have probably been content with blood glucose levels that are higher than normal. If they follow the program outlined here, they could be enjoying blood glucose readings in the normal range.

When you begin this program, there will be some obvious hurdles to overcome. Some hurdles will be higher than others, depending on the nature of your diabetes when the condition was diagnosed and that all-important, irreplaceable component, your attitude. Yes, it will be tough for you to give up certain beloved foods, at least for a while. More formidable may be the resistance you encounter from your doctor (if he or she is not on the cutting edge of current research on the subject), family, and friends, and other diabetics who are still wedded to the old way. But rest assured that respected endocrinologists and diabetologists who are ahead of the curve now advocate similar diet and exercise guidelines. And rest assured that using this program will put you on the right path toward a consistently normal blood sugar and away from the complications that result when blood sugar is not well controlled. Of course, no one should try the plan without being under a doctor's care. That's what I've done, and the program has worked for me. Who knows? The results you get may even change your own doctor's way of thinking and contribute to the wellness of other diabetics.

Think of this book as a travel guide to one of the most common yet least visited medical countries in the world of disease and aging. This guide will help you read the road signs, choose the rest stops, and find the best route for you to successful treatment and the prevention of complications. It will make you feel up to the task of charting your own course and reduce the fears that can arise from all the conflicting and sometimes misleading information you are about to receive from the medical profession and well-meaning friends and family. Enjoy your trip. It will be illuminating, and it can improve your life.

What I learned in my travels through all the conflicting information and conflicting treatment recommendations for diabetes is this: Each of us is the best master of his or her diabetes treatment. And another wonderfully kept secret in the confusing maze of diabetes information is that unless a person with diabetes is on his or her deathbed, he or she *can* do better. It may be only a little bit better at first, but the positive effects of your nutrition and exercise regime can be cumulative—and over time, a little bit better can become a lot.

Managing diabetes means working on a puzzle composed of many intricate pieces. It is a challenging puzzle, one you'll have to concentrate on. Now and then a piece will confound you, and you'll have to try it again in different ways in different places. But it is also a fascinating puzzle, one that will hold your interest because it is about you, the hero of your own story, and about making your life a better place and improving your capacity to enjoy that life. As long as you persevere and are patient, you will be able to solve the puzzle and see the big picture, because with the help of this book, your doctor, and your support team, you have all the pieces you need to complete the puzzle.

ABOUT DIABETES AND DRUGS

Many more Type II diabetics could manage their diabetes without the aid of oral hypoglycemic agents (OHAs) if they managed good control of blood glucose levels with diet and exercise. *Beat Diabetes!* is geared to helping those who can manage without OHAs or with less medication, whether it be OHAs or insulin. However, this is not a treatise on avoiding insulin and OHAs at all costs. Rather, it is an affirmation of the new "big picture" for diabetics. The current overview is that almost all of us have the possibility of keeping blood sugar in the normal range with the right individualized treatment. In that light, the program can maintain your blood glucose readings in the normal range. It can keep you in good overall health whether or not you need to add medication to your treatment regimen. In the end, there is no getting around the ultimate truth that the underpinning of any successful treatment for diabetes is a diet and exercise regimen that helps regulate blood glucose levels.

All of us must manage diabetes as well as she or he can. (And I know and appreciate that how much you can do and will do varies from person to person.) As you read this book, keep in mind that what may have worked for me may not work for everyone else. One diabetic's healthy regimen may be another diabetic's blood glucose nightmare.

What do I mean by "managing your diabetes as well as you can"? I mean maintaining consistently normal blood glucose levels. If you cannot do this without taking medication, by all means you should take medication—but the right kind and the right dose (see If You Are Taking Insulin or OHAs). This doesn't mean you've failed; it means that taking medication is the course you need to take to succeed. Diabetes is a case where the means do justify the end—the end being controlling your blood sugar.

If you do take insulin or oral medication to help manage your diabetes, however, you cannot allow yourself to use this as an excuse to lead a gustatory life filled with tortilla chips and ice cream sundaes or pasta and rice. The era of the high-carbohydrate diet for diabetics is on its way out, finally and for the good of all of us. A diet laden in carbohydrates, even complex carbohydrates, is the road to disaster. The cardinal rule of diabetes treatment is that what you put into your mouth will directly affect your blood sugar. Both Type I and Type II diabetics will benefit from the low-carbohydrate, high-protein, and exercise-intensive program outlined in this book; it will help all diabetics get in good shape and normalize blood sugar, as long as they are under a doctor's care and using medication if they need to.

If you are taking insulin, you'll want to modify your diet so that what you eat and when you eat it works in tandem with your insulin injections. An excellent guide in helping you make those alterations is *Dr. Bernstein's Diabetes Solution*.

HOW I BEAT DIABETES

My case is paradigmatic of the ongoing debate over how to define and treat diabetes. And had I listened to the powers that be, I would be a drug-dependent diabetic whose risk of complications would be increasing every year.

As a medical writer, I'd had enough experience with the medical profession to understand that the time to ask questions about your treatment is before it starts. I researched the subject on my own so that I would know what questions to ask. I found experts who dared to challenge the status quo.

In the process, I examined the facts: I was not a brittle diabetic with no insulin production at all; my pancreas was still producing the hormone, albeit in less than normal amounts. And then I isolated the problem: how to maximize the efficiency of the insulin my system had available to it by minimizing the amount of carbohydrate it had to process. I now manage Type I diabetes without drugs, controlling my blood glucose levels and keeping them in the mid to low range of normal with diet and exercise. This equation of diet and exercise, plus perseverance, offers nearly miraculous results and could change the lives of thousands of diabetics—indeed, it could save the lives of many. In the literature on diabetes, the patient's story gets short shrift. I know how hard it is because I've done it. I know all the caveats of human fallibility and implementation. I know we fall from grace and have to rise above a lot of negative impulses. And I know nobody's perfect, because I'm not. So you can trust me when I say that what I have to share with other diabetics is a plan that has worked for me, keeps on working for me, and has improved my general health and my life (without turning me into a saint, I might add).

IF A TREE FALLS IN THE FOREST . . .

Implemented successfully, the program in *Beat Diabetes!* creates a welcome paradox of diagnosis: A diabetic with blood glucose levels consistently in the normal range is not a diabetic. Through establishing this diet and exercise regimen, many diabetics cannot cure the disease, but they can stay in recovery for life (to borrow a term from the alcohol and drug treatment world). Interestingly, the longer a diabetic maintains the program, the more efficient the pancreas becomes at producing the necessary insulin—thus effectively "healing" itself, to a partial extent.

In the case of diabetes, the adage "blood will tell" is particularly apposite. Testing your blood lets you know when you're on the right course and when you're going wrong. Your blood testing kit is your compass, helping you chart a healthy course. Normal mid-range blood glucose levels are all the proof you need that you are going in the right direction. Being diagnosed with diabetes is not the terrible life sentence it once was. *Beat Diabetes!* will help those diagnosed with diabetes see the diagnosis as a turning point on the road to better health, a milestone that marks the beginning of a better life.

A NON-DISCLAIMER

If you have diabetes or know you are at risk for diabetes, I hope that this will not be the only book you read on the subject. If you are a long-term Type I diabetic or even a late onset Type I diabetic, this book may not be for you; it might be too relaxed in its approach to what Dr. Richard Bernstein calls "immaculate care." Immaculate care refers to maintaining nearly perfect control of blood glucose levels with an extremely restricted diet and an intensively monitored insulin regimen.

It does work for me, however, and I'm generally considered a late onset Type I diabetic. Then again, I may be a lean Type II diabetic—not even her diabetologists know for sure! You see, everything really is topsy turvey in the world of diabetes. Rather than being a "downer" for diabetics, the state of flux in the study of diabetes augers well for better treatment for all of us. At this point, the one thing all my various doctors agree on is that if I can keep blood glucose levels normal without ruining my health in other ways, I don't need drugs. So, don't call me Type I or Type II, just call me non-insulin dependent. Definitions are changing, and treatment is changing. It bodes well for all of us.

This is not a cookbook, an exercise manual, or even a memoir. It's a book to get you started, inspire you, and keep you keeping at it. It won't drive you away by setting impossible goals or asking you to do impossible math or act as if you're not human. To be human is to be prone to lapses of all kinds. What you need most is not a punishing program or a "hair shirt" made up of rules and regulations. What you need is a simple and practical program to keep you inspired—if you want to live well with diabetes.

That's what I'm doing—living well with diabetes, not fighting against it. That's what I want for you. And living well with diabetes is easier than all the piles of information you already have on the subject lead you to believe.

FARE FORWARD VOYAGER

I know that when you read this program, it will sound grueling at first. I know you'll be asking, "How will I have time to live my life if it takes this much time to manage my diabetes?" I know you're already asking yourself, "Is it worth it?" Well, it is, for a number of reasons:

- What you do now to control your diabetes will help ensure that you don't have to cope with complications later and that you live a long and healthy life.
- When you use this diet and exercise plan to control your blood sugar, you also protect yourself against a host of other diseases for which we are all at greater risk as we age, including heart disease, stroke, certain forms of cancer, and even osteoporosis (your anaerobic weight routine will help build strong bones as well as burn glucose).
- You will feel better. You will have more energy and more enthusiasm for the things you want to do. The lethargy that many of us assume is a normal part of the aging process will lift. Feeling better is inarguable. (I am now 44, and I feel younger than I did when I was 36. Believe me, it's worth it.)

- You will be surprised at just how quickly your new routine becomes a way of life. Soon you'll be saying, "It's second nature to me now," and as you begin to feel better, you'll become even more dedicated to your new way of life. And in the maelstrom of modern life, you may even feel comforted by the actions you take daily to take care of yourself. No matter what happens, no matter what life has in store for you, taking care of your health will be your port in the storm.

I worry that because I was diagnosed early, some readers may think this book is not for them—you know, the "I only wish *I'd* been so lucky . . . " syndrome. In "shrinkeze," this is called a rationalization. Wherever you are on the continuum of diabetes, there is something in this book that can help you. I may have been diagnosed "in time" (before my blood sugar hit 500 mg/dL), but whenever you start, you can turn back the hands of diabetes, as long as you stick to it. I know how hard it can be for any diabetic to cope, and I know that diet and exercise do make all the difference, especially when combined with a positive attitude. (Sorry, but Pollyanna did have a few things right.) Read on—because you can do it too!

part 1
Welcome to My Pancreas

Diabetes has been around for centuries. Until the twentieth century and the advent of insulin therapy, it was a not so silent killer. That diabetes was for most of history a terminal disease is part of the reason for its terrible reputation.

Even though progress has been made, I was not surprised to hear on a national news program that diabetes is "a silent killer" that "creeps up slowly over time." Well, if this helps people, fine. The truth is that it creeps up over a long period of time and that doctors should be responsible for monitoring patients' blood sugars over time. Then, believe me, it will not creep up. The problems can be solved before they begin. I'm not absolving the patients. Probably the worst thing that occurs when diabetes is diagnosed is that patients feel defeated and don't try. But almost equally appalling is that diabetes is not diagnosed when it ought to be—early, when you can change your life, when there is hope, when you have a very good chance of leading a normal life.

Though attitudes are changing, the disease is still inadequately treated with the available drugs. Patients are often overtreated or not treated at all—an estimated five million Americans do not even know they have the disease. Finally, however, advances in medical technology, medication, and the new emphasis on exercise and the evolving diabetic diet are beginning to improve the outlook and the quality of life for most diabetics, and increase life expectancy as well.

It's about time. While estimates vary, the number of diabetics in the United States is approximately sixteen million or more, and that number is on the rise. In the past thirty years in the United States, the number of diabetics has risen by 700 percent.

(Guess why? The reason is because of a sedentary lifestyle and obesity.) Even more alarming, young adults are now being diagnosed with Type II diabetes.

We should all be shocked by this. Unfortunately, few who have political clout and hold the purse strings have been. In addition, every 60 seconds at least one more American is diagnosed with diabetes. This year alone more than half a million people will be diagnosed with the disease. In addition, each year over 160,000 Americans die from the disease and its complications, more than the number who die from breast cancer or lung cancer. And by the year 2000, it is estimated that a staggering one-tenth of all Americans will have diabetes. And diabetes is a major global health problem as well. According to the International Diabetes Federation, an estimated one hundred million people worldwide are afflicted with this disease. If these numbers are not enough to spur further research toward more effective treatments and a cure, perhaps calling attention to the dent in America's pocket caused by the disease will do the trick. The yearly cost of diabetes to the United States is $100 billion. It's time.

1

A Diabetes Primer

A diagnosis of diabetes resembles a confusing nightmare, where all kinds of new terms are introduced and talk of blood and needles begins. It can be hard to keep the subtle differences in nomenclature straight and to keep your own fears under control. Therefore, before we discuss the program that will change your life, let's address how the disease is currently classified and treated.

Diabetes mellitus is a disorder of the endocrine system—an elegant and complex network of interacting glands or glandular tissue that secrete hormones, the body's chemical messengers. Hormones act much like maestros, each conducting, controlling, and regulating a particular bodily function. From "pianissimo" to "forte," variations in the amount of the hormone make a great deal of difference in the performance. Almost every organ of the body is affected by our hormones, which regulate functions as diverse as growth, metabolism, maintenance of the body's fluid balance, and reproduction. Like any orchestra, the organs of the body would be bewildered and out of synch without hormonal leadership. Our hormones also allow the body to react protectively to internal and external stimuli in the environment.

Diabetes could be called an umbrella term for a range of conditions that affect blood sugar, but in general, diabetics are classified as either Type I or Type II diabetics. Type I diabetes used to be called juvenile onset diabetes because most of those diagnosed with it get the disease before they are in their twenties. Type II diabetes was called adult onset diabetes. Type I diabetes may also be referred to as IDDM (insulin dependent diabetes mellitus), and Type II diabetes as NIDDM (non-insulin dependent diabetes mellitus). Though as mentioned in the introduction, many Type II diabetics may become insulin dependent. This is evidence of the shifting sands when it comes to defining and treating diabetes.

Beyond these names, the way in which the two types of diabetes are distinguished from each other can vary considerably. (This is evidence of how little we actually understand the disease.) What distinguishes Type I from Type II diabetes is the lack of insulin production. A Type I diabetic has a pancreas that produces less insulin than a normal pancreas or no insulin at all—those in the latter condition are designated as *brittle* diabetics. By contrast, the pancreas of a Type II diabetic still produces insulin, but the person's body has become resistant to that insulin, usually because of obesity. In other words, in Type I diabetics, there isn't enough insulin to go around, and in Type II diabetics, insulin is prevented from doing its designated job well. To reiterate, a Type II diabetic can do so much damage to his or her pancreas with poor control that he or she may eventually become insulin dependent—for all intents and purposes a Type I diabetic, though the diabetic in question may not be defined that way. (It should be noted, however, that these distinctions vary from text to text. Sometimes they are blurred, and sometimes they are even contradictory, which increases the confusion that surrounds diabetes—who gets it, when and why, and how to treat it.)

Confusion also surrounds the treatment of the disease, and this confusion contributes to the mistreatment of many diabetics—one that exacts a heavy price in often lethal complications. Most doctors believe that the best way— indeed the only way—to treat diabetes is with insulin injections (in the case of Type I diabetics) or with oral agents (Type II diabetics). The assumption is that prevention and early intervention are not worthwhile, in fact, not even possible. The overtreatment of diabetes has become a medical habit.

Diabetes has been recognized as an illness since antiquity. The term *diabetes mellitus* was coined by the Greeks, and references to diabetes occur as early as 1500 B.C. *Diabetes* means "to siphon or pass through," which refers to the common symptom of copious urination in untreated diabetics. Samuel Johnson defined diabetes as "a morbid copiousness of urine; a fatal colliquation by the urinary passages." Early physicians also noticed that the urine of a diabetic had a sweet odor—ergo, *mellitus,* the Latin word for honey. This happens because glucose (a sugar) builds up in the blood over time, and eventually some of it spills over into the urine. In fact, early tests for diabetes involved smelling and often tasting the urine for sweetness. To this day, many diabetics are diagnosed after a routine urinalysis indicates sugar in the urine.

In his highly praised, *Natural Health, Natural Medicine*, Dr. Andrew Weil evinces the hypothesis that diabetes may have been an adaptive trait at one time in human history. For thousands of years, the human diet consisted mainly of complex carbohydrates from raw fruits and vegetables and plenty of protein from meat and other animal products (though Dr. Weil is not so keen on this component of our ancestors' diet)—a diet that keeps blood glucose levels naturally low. And, of course, in early hunter-gatherer societies, people automatically led nonsedentary lives. The level of activity was strenuous but steady, over periods of time that were long in duration—a much better workout for a diabetic than a short, intense one.

The earliest form of metabolism was glycolysis. In this process, after an extensive period of aerobic exercise, oxygen is no longer able to reach the muscle cells in sufficient quantity. The supply of glucose used for energy is exhausted, and enzymes in the muscle cells cut glucose (glycolysize it) in order to supply the cells with energy. (This is a perfect health and fitness scenario for a diabetic.) The daily routine of hunter-gatherers also included anaerobic exercise—the lifting and carrying of weights, in this case, tribal possessions or the "kill"—another important factor in keeping glucose levels low.

Weil's theory that producing less insulin (because less insulin was necessary to regulate blood glucose) probably has some validity. It is indeed possible to regard diabetes as a disease of civilization. Certainly, it is far more prevalent in cultures with a sedentary lifestyle and a high occurrence of obesity, such as the United States, than it is in cultures where people work outdoors and eat few processed fats, fast foods, junk foods, and simple carbohydrates, such as French fries and pizza.

Among the most important hormones in the endocrine system's chemical arsenal is insulin. It's one of three hormones that until recently were considered to be the only hormones produced by the pancreas (see And What About the Future?). The other two are glucagon, which breaks down the glucose that is stored in the liver as glycogen, and somatostatin, which seems to be important in regulating both production and release of insulin and glucagon (although its role is still unclear, and further research may offer more information on how this hormone affects the role of insulin). Insulin is produced in tiny clusters of pancreatic cells called the islets of Langerhans, a poetic name for a production plant. The islets of Langerhans contain both alpha cells and beta cells. Glucagon is released by the alpha cells.

Insulin is released by the beta cells. These hormones enable the body to turn food into fuel. When the beta cells are damaged, as in Type I diabetes, and the pancreas produces little or no insulin, the efficient manufacturing and distribution of fuel (in the form of glucose) is jeopardized. When a person is obese and the pancreas is called upon to produce more and more insulin in order to process the glucose offered by such large amounts of food, as in Type II diabetes, insulin resistance occurs. The body becomes inured to this life-sustaining hormone. In both cases, diabetes is the result.

Before the 1920s, a diabetic whose pancreas could not produce insulin lived no more than 10 years after the diagnosis, and children diagnosed with diabetes lived only a matter of months. In 1921, Dr. Charles Best and Dr. Frederick Banting extracted a substance (later identified as insulin) from a cow's pancreas and injected it into a diabetic dog. Almost immediately, the dog's blood sugar was lowered. The discovery of insulin therapy caused a revolution in diabetes treatment almost overnight, offering diabetics a life with a future, if not a cure. Insulin was heralded as a wonder drug—more correctly a wonder replacement hormone. But insulin does not solve all of the problems of a diabetic: Injecting it creates new problems even as it solves the primary one of lack of insulin production. In particular, an injection of a high dose of insulin demands an immediate supply of carbohydrate to give the insulin something to "feed" on and to avoid exceedingly low blood sugars—hypoglycemia—which can be as dangerous to the diabetic as hyperglycemia (high blood sugar).

Two out of three diabetics are from families where there is some history of diabetes, but genetic proclivity alone does not determine that a person will become diabetic. Other factors, particularly lifestyle and the effects of viral infections on the beta cells of the pancreas, are also important pieces in the puzzle of diabetes. Although in some cases Type I diabetes develops suddenly, for the most part, diabetes is a slow onset condition. And speculation that a viral infection may cause the immune system to misfire and destroy beta cells in its quest to eradicate the invading virus may also place diabetes in the ever-increasing realm of autoimmune-related diseases.

2

Being Diagnosed

Someone who is diagnosed with diabetes later in life usually has some warning signs, not the least of which may be a blood glucose reading at the high end of normal at more than one physical checkup (see Warning Signs and Symptoms; and Risk Factors). Still, even if you think you are prepared to hear the news, you're never really prepared. I know because that's what happened to me.

In 1989, during a routine, prenatal checkup, my doctor found that sugar had spilled into my urine. I went for a glucose tolerance test, and, sure enough, I had gestational diabetes. In one week, I managed to normalize my blood sugar by eliminating all fruit juice from my diet and switching to a diet composed mainly of fresh vegetables and protein, including my daily quart of milk for calcium. (If I had known that milk is higher in carbohydrate value than cream or cheese or yogurt, I would have gotten my calcium elsewhere. Still, for the standards of treatment of the day, I did pretty well.) I don't have a sweet tooth, so giving up desserts wasn't much of an issue.

The medical party line was that my blood glucose levels would "go back to normal" as soon as I gave birth. Of course, nothing went back to normal after I gave birth, including my blood sugar levels. Everything had changed. And at every checkup thereafter, my doctor—who is one of the few doctors who does pay close attention to blood glucose levels at checkups—always noted that my blood sugar always ran a little high, at the outside edge of what was then considered normal.

Warning Signs and Symptoms

There are many warning signs and symptoms for diabetes, if you are willing to heed them. Here is the quartet of symptoms: excessive (even insatiable) thirst, frequent urination, sudden weight loss, unusual hunger.

If your blood glucose levels have been high for a long period of time, you may also experience fatigue, nausea and vomiting, skin infections, bladder infections, and blurred vision. Women may have frequent bouts with vaginitis and men may experience impotence. If you are experiencing such symptoms, technically you have probably had diabetes for a while.

The trick is to discover that you have diabetes before you have any of these symptoms so that you can begin to treat the disease and normalize blood sugar before any permanent damage has occurred (see Risk Factors).

If you do notice that you are thirsty, urinating often, and/or losing weight suddenly, even though your appetite has increased, you should see your doctor for a blood test. Avoiding a diagnosis of diabetes is fool's gold. The longer you avoid the news, the greater your risk of complications and the more difficult your diabetes will be to treat.

The information given to pregnant women about gestational diabetes is minimal and often confusing. It is generally agreed, however, that approximately 50 to 60 percent of all women who develop gestational diabetes will develop diabetes permanently within the next 10 years. This percentage is alarmingly high, and yet new mothers who had gestational diabetes are given no counseling regarding how to avoid diabetes in the future, nor is screening with routine blood tests recommended to them. Originally it was thought that these women eventually developed Type II diabetes, but recent research indicates that women who've had gestational diabetes generally develop Type I diabetes and eventually become insulin dependent.

As a medical writer, I was aware that more than half the women who have diabetes when pregnant end up with diabetes in the long run, and with this in mind, I monitored my condition with the help of my doctor and doing the best I could on the old carbohydrate diet coupled with a rigorous aerobic exercise routine. I was fortunate that I had a wonderful internist in New York City. His offices were literally on the street where I lived, and while we didn't fall in love or sing romantic musical standards to each other, I do credit him with the kind of medical care most people only dream of finding (probably a rarer occurrence than finding someone to sing ballads with). That Dr. Martin Beitler is my doctor is also one of the few things I have my ex-husband to thank for. He, my ex-husband, arrived home at the loft one evening, where I was nursing our son and trying to cook dinner, saying, "There's this new doctor at Spring and Greene Street. He takes Oxford. We're going to him." And go we did. Marriage and divorce work in strange ways. You never know what you're going to end up grateful for.

At 36, I didn't have that many aches and pains, but I had some. I was also conscientious about going for my yearly physical, particularly because I had begun a new career as a medical writer and felt I would be a terrible hypocrite if I didn't do at least some of the wise things I preached. Each year that I went for my physical, Dr. Beitler would say, "Well, your blood glucose is 116mg/dL. That's a little high for me. We'll have to watch it." Such an approach wasn't revolutionary, but in the early 1990s, there were not many internists routinely reporting on your blood glucose levels and calling borderline normal readings something to watch. I was lucky.

I was also a somewhat more informed candidate for diabetes than some. And I liked to cook. I joked that you didn't have to wear Birkenstocks to grind your own oats and make your own baby food. I was a full-time mother and a full-time writer. On a daily basis, there was pureed yellow split pea soup in the keyboard, and my son's head was propped on a hand that held a draft of this or that for my perusal while he nursed. I was in the habit of cooking healthy meals for my husband and myself. These were low-fat meals, since the "hands-on" Dr. Beitler had warned my husband that his cholesterol level was getting too high.

With the help of a friend who worked at my favorite organic foods store, I started to incorporate more complex carbohydrates

Risk Factors

If you are over 40 and your doctor does not mention your blood glucose level at your yearly checkup, ask him or her to. As we age, everyone is at higher risk for diabetes, just as we are for heart disease. Approximately 80 percent of newly diagnosed Type II diabetics are over 40. Type I diabetics are generally diagnosed before the age of 30; and males are most often diagnosed between the ages of 12 and 14, and females are most often diagnosed between the ages of 10 and 12.

If you have a family history of the disease, your risk of developing Type II diabetes is much greater. If you have an identical twin with Type II diabetes, there is nearly a 100 percent chance that you will develop diabetes. Type I diabetes also clusters in families, but not as Type II diabetes.

Being overweight is an extremely strong risk factor for Type II diabetes. At least 80 percent of people with Type II diabetes weigh at least 20 percent more than their ideal weight. Weight is not a risk factor for Type I diabetes. If you are overweight, you should try to lose weight.

If you have had gestational diabetes, you are more than twice as likely to develop diabetes within the next 10 years. Most women who have had gestational diabetes develop Type II diabetes, but it is possible to develop Type I diabetes after having gestational diabetes. If you have had gestational diabetes and have not yet developed Type II diabetes, you should monitor your blood glucose levels with your doctor and follow the diet and exercise plan outlined in this book (see Understanding Gestational Diabetes).

Some researchers believe that a faulty immune system may be a factor in causing Type I diabetes. The theory is that an infection of the pancreas may, in effect, cause the immune system to

into our diet to work toward lowering my blood glucose levels as well as my husband's cholesterol. Call it a contrapuntal dance of the diets. This friend was also studying biochemistry, and he was most helpful in describing that I needed to eat small meals and give my system complex carbohydrates, which take time to digest and, therefore, don't call for sudden spurts of insulin but rather smaller amounts of insulin over time. I was doing pretty well.

Then what had always been a difficult marriage began to escalate into something more. By the beginning of the winter of 1994–95, I was under tremendous stress. While I coped

backfire and destroy the beta cells in the pancreas that produce insulin. This theory of metabolic self-destruction gains support because Type I diabetes is often diagnosed after a bout with the flu, chickenpox, or even a bad cold. The antibodies of the immune system designed to attack beta cells can often be found in the blood of those who develop Type I diabetes.

Environmental factors may also increase your risk for Type II diabetes. In other words, a sedentary lifestyle and a diet filled with starches are a potent combination that will increase your risk dramatically.

Race is a strong risk factor for Type II diabetes. Between the ages of 45 and 55, approximately twice as many African-Americans as white Americans have diabetes. Native-Americans have twice the risk of developing Type II diabetes as white

Americans, and Mexican-Americans have three times the risk of developing the disease.

Race is also a contributing risk factor for Type I diabetes. The highest incidence of Type I diabetes occurs among people of Scandinavian descent.

Anyone in these categories should take the precaution of having their fasting blood glucose level checked at their yearly physical. The new guidelines indicate that a fasting blood level of 126mg/dL or higher is now a sign of diabetes, as opposed to the old number of 140mg/dL. In fact, all older Americans should have their blood glucose level checked on a yearly basis. In the past, the urine was tested for any spills of sugar into the urine, but the truth is, that by the time sugar spills into the urine, blood glucose levels are quite high and have been elevated for a long period of time.

well and had many friends and a rugged sense of mental and emotional balance (I had to keep it together—I had a son), the situation did begin to take its toll on my physical health. The pressure I lived with didn't give me much of an appetite, and gradually my healthy habits deteriorated, not a lot, but enough.

After my son and I moved out (my husband would not budge), my financial burdens were even greater. Thus, while I had put distance between myself and a very stressful relationship, I'd added other stresses to my life. Things settled down. Life went on. I took writer-for-hire jobs, working harder and harder, enjoying my son, but a bit the worse for wear. Then, the following winter of 1995–96—the winter of the blizzards—I was diagnosed with diabetes. The "you-know-what" does always hit the fan eventually.

I got the news from Dr. Beitler on a Monday afternoon, shortly before I had to pick up my son from school. Dr. B. looked at the results of my blood work for that year's checkup, and said, "Well, your fasting blood was 140. That's diabetes. It's time for an oral agent."

"It's time? Just like that?" I asked. "Give me a moment." Here I was trying to chew on my tongue to keep from crying, and here he was perfunctorily prescribing—his job, of course, but the job of the patient is to question until they understand. The more we participate in our treatment, the more likely that treatment is to succeed.

This diagnosis was no surprise, right? I was "Miss Enlightenment" when it came to diabetes, right? Not so right. Even with all my knowledge and preparation, it came as a surprise just the same. No matter how much we prepare, a piece of bad news is a shock when it comes. I was as traumatized by the news as if I had been ignorant of the possibility in the first place.

The American Diabetes New Guidelines

In an article in the New York Times on June 24, 1997, it was reported that according to the American Diabetes New Guidelines, millions of Americans who have not been tested for diabetes need to be tested. When I read the article, I really wanted to say, "I told you so" to someone, but then I thought, well at least we are finally giving diabetes the attention it deserves and should have been getting years ago. Good news is still good news, even if it comes a little late.

According to the new guidelines, a person with a blood sugar level of 126 mg/dL is considered to have provisional diabetes. A person with a blood glucose level of 110 to 125mg/dL is considered to be impaired, and blood glucose levels under 110 mg/dL are considered normal.

These guidelines are a far cry from the old ones. In the old days, you weren't considered to be diabetic unless your blood glucose levels were 140 mg/dLs or above. And that's not all; the ADA guidelines also state that everyone over 45 should be tested routinely for diabetes. In addition, it recommends that anyone with high cholesterol levels or high blood pressure be tested frequently, as well as those in other high-risk groups. These groups include anyone with a relative who has diabetes, anyone who is obese (more than 20 percent overweight), women who've had gestational diabetes, African Americans, Hispanics, and Native Americans, and finally, anyone who has had impaired glucose tolerance on previous testing.

Finally, the country has gotten the wake-up call.

IN SEARCH OF
THE RIGHT TREATMENT

I love my doctor, but—as he would be the first to tell you—diabetes is not ultimately his specialty. Doctors assume that anyone diagnosed over the age of 40 is a Type II diabetic, and oral agents, which combat the insulin resistance characteristic of Type II, are almost always the treatment of choice. But I was still absorbing the new information and I knew that I needed even more. I bargained with my doctor for another week. He agreed. The events of the next few days would prove the wisdom of not beginning oral agents right away.

I left his office to pick up my son at school. I kept thinking that my life had changed irrevocably, but it hadn't changed at all.

Through a close friend, I obtained an appointment with Dr. Bernstein, the guru of the diabetes revolution, who has popularized and who champions the concept of "tight control"—keeping blood glucose levels and minimizing amplitude—in diabetes treatment. I went armed with all the information I could muster on the subject, knowing that it is incumbent upon the patient to be able to ask the right questions as well as understand the answers that doctors often couch in daunting and obscure terms. I wanted to be able to be my own interpreter when confronted with the foreign language doctors so often use.

The day of my appointment, I took the train from Grand Central Station to suburban Mamaroneck, where Dr. Bernstein has his offices, feeling if not positive at least composed and resigned. I could manage Type II diabetes. I exercised. I ate a healthy diet. I was slim. If I had to do more, I could and I would. Though I was on the low end of the weight curve and the high end of the curve for informed self-care, it never crossed my mind that I was dealing with anything but Type II diabetes and insulin resistance.

To my surprise, it did cross Dr. Bernstein's mind. He looked at me. He looked at my fasting blood glucose in my medical records and said, "You're probably Type I." I cringed, thinking in as stereotypic fashion as the next non-diabetic, "Type I, the kind with the shots."

Sure enough, the next thing he said was, "I think we should get you on insulin right away to give your pancreas a rest."

I'd come to see this specialist for a strategy, but not this one. I stiffened.

"What's the matter?" he asked. "You worried about the shot?"

"No. It's the concept," I said.

"Here, let me show you," he said, and he took a small, plastic disposable syringe from its wrapper and came around the desk. After a short debate, I held out my arm, and he stuck the needle through the sleeve of my white turtleneck just like that. It was fast and painless, and there was no blood—a very neat job, all in all. But I was not convinced. "I came here for your wonder diet. I can get insulin anywhere."

Now, I found myself bargaining with another doctor for another week. We fashioned a daily meal plan that included only 30 grams of carbohydrates, none of them from grains or other staples of the low-fat diet so in vogue. I had to give up pasta, breads, rice, soups and stews, grains, legumes, and fruits. What I couldn't eat could fill a book. What I could eat wouldn't fill one page: protein (including meat, fish, eggs and cheese), salad (with no tomatoes and with oil and vinegar), and most green vegetables, as long as they were not overcooked. The plan looked grim. I had a strange sensation of being the carrier of my own plague. Life's a prison, sure, but then sometimes the bars are a little more real than others. This was one of those times. I could run, but I couldn't hide. (I wasn't supposed to run anyway, unless I wanted to run a marathon. Aerobic activity over short periods of time can raise blood glucose levels. Anaerobic or static activity, which involves weight resistance, can burn glucose . . . but I'm getting ahead of myself.) I felt trapped. I was glad to get out of there and get busy eating, or not eating, running, or not running. A clinical setting makes any condition seem worse.

I had my second appointment with Dr. Bernstein the very next morning, returning to have him do my blood work personally. (He's careful about labs and wanted to use his own lab rather than trust the lab my internist uses.) As he had done the day before, he tested my blood glucose level on his own Glucometer (with a fresh lancet—the tiny needle that pricks your finger, thank you). The reading was 20 points lower than the day before at approximately the same time of day. Despite that bit of good news, he told me he wanted me to give myself a shot. I was quite surprised, and I was all for putting it off, but he was concerned about an infection. If I needed insulin immediately because of an infection, he wanted to be able to prescribe it over the phone. (When he explained to me that a diabetic's blood glucose levels may rise dramatically due to a common cold, virus, or, for that matter, any infection and cause further damage to the pancreas, I was all in favor of knowing how to give myself the shot in an emergency.) And since there was no cajoling him out of this second act with a needle anyway, I decided I wanted to do a good job giving myself the shot. I managed on the first try, with commendations from the doctor.

When I picked up my son and a friend from school that afternoon, it was snowing and there was already 6 inches on the ground. After a few snowballs, I took them, laughing and running (not me, them), to the local drugstore, where I bought my Glucometer (and a plastic action figure for each of them). The advent of the Glucometer has also been essential to the revolution in diabetes care. Insert a test strip, prick your finger with the automatically controlled lancet, apply a drop of blood to the test strip, and in 60 seconds you know your blood glucose level. It is this instrument that allows diabetics to control their health in a way that was impossible earlier in medical history—providing, of course, that they are willing to take the matter of personal health literally into their own hands.

That afternoon at home, I pricked my finger with the lancet for the first time. My blood glucose was 112 mg/dL, almost normal. I was elated. Mid-range normal blood glucose is between 85 and 95 mg/dL, and normal blood glucose is considered to run between 80 and 110 to 116 mg/dL, depending on the lab.

By the end of a week, my fingers were riddled with tiny pin-pricks, but it was worth it. My readings were consistently between 77 and 115 mg/dL, except when I exercised. The elevated readings after my aerobic exercise routine stood out like a sore thumb each day. They were proof positive that as good as aerobic exercise may be for everything else, aerobic exercise must be handled carefully by the diabetic.

Anaerobic exercise seemed to be the only way to go. Dr. Bernstein had told me and I'd read that it burned eighteen times the glucose of aerobic activity. Now, I have always found weight lifting a peculiar activity—nothing against Arnold Schwarzenegger. But if this was the kind of exercise that was going to help me now, then you can bet I'd at least try to pump iron with the best of them. The first couple of times I pumped iron my readings were steady, which was good enough. Soon, they began to descend—not a lot, but enough to make me a convert. Now I do a weight training routine every day. I also walk between 5 and 6 miles a day in an effort to take care of the health of my heart. In addition, now that my blood glucose levels have normalized, I've added aerobic exercise to my life once again, with no ill effects (see The Sisyphus Strategy: Lift Weights, Walk Uphill, Don't Stop).

For once in my addled life, things worked well. I kept a log of blood glucose levels—recording them six times a day and faxing them to my doctor over a 2-week period. We touched base each week. He was impressed. At the end of the 2 weeks, he told me, "You're remarkable and remarkably easy to manage." So far, so good.

I was motivated by Dr. Bernstein's logic, by his precise planning, and by the specter of that needle with which I shadow-boxed daily. (I don't mean to be anti-insulin or politically incorrect. I admire every diabetic who uses insulin and manages all the details of such a regimen in addition to the rest of the daily demands of life. I can only hope I could do as well as my friends who cope with the adding, subtracting, remembering, and injecting.) I knew that if I had to, I'd use the tiny needle and the milky, white liquid it delivered. I'd cope with needing insulin because a Pyrrhic victory can kill you. But in the beginning, I let keeping the specter at bay motivate me. As time wore on, however, and I worked out the kinks of my personal resistance and daily life's little whirlwinds, I began to be motivated by the game itself. I saw each day as an experiment, a unit of time in which to explore the best combination of the variables of diet and exercise into an equation that would end up equaling a blood sugar reading in the normal range and without any dramatic spiking up or down.

Mostly I found that when it comes to being diagnosed—attitude is everything. Hang in there. Your moodiness will pass. Get help. Get comfort. Then get to work.

THE LONG AND WINDING ROAD

Guess what? This was not the end of my diagnostic journey. In fact, it was only the beginning of my trip through the funhouse of diagnoses, semi-diagnoses, and misdiagnoses. For some time, I did the mild Type I/lean Type II rag with my doctor. Then we did the Type I foxtrot. Every time I had a cold or the flu or other infection, I was definitely Type I and "cruisin' for a bruisin'" if I didn't shoot up insulin. Then, when my change in diet so immediately enhanced my blood glucose readings, we were back to the Type I/Type II rag, and on and on. This was a shadow dance, but as long as I was keeping the bgs in normal range, who cared? Not me. (I never did like the Bee Gees. So who wanted to give them any higher rating numbers?)

Eventually, both Dr. Bernstein and I agreed that I could manage my condition more conveniently and at less cost by seeing an associate of his in New York City.

HYPOCHONDRIAC'S DELIGHT

In addition to feeling overwhelmed and as if everything but the kitchen sink had been dumped on my head, the kitchen sink finally hit me too—in the form of a rampant case of hypochondria. It was as if all those minor hypochondriac fantasies inspired by years of medical writing finally had a real focus, and boy did they come out of the woodwork.

If my hands were numb on a subzero day, I prophesied neuropathy. If I squinted to read a newspaper, I predicted eventual blindness. If my period was a day late, I was sure I was experiencing dysmenorrhea, a rare symptom in advanced cases of diabetes. The stress I was causing myself over my closet full of complications was surely raising my blood glucose levels, but still I kept gnattering at myself like a mad woodpecker at a tree.

And I didn't have to look into the proverbial handful of dust to see my fear. I saw infection everywhere, saw my own fear in every scrape or cut. I was a hypochondriac set loose in the infectious diseases unit, to say nothing of the diabetic in a candy store. I had available to me the lure and propaganda of the well-advertised complications of diabetes and the knowledge that an infection may damage the pancreas further and drive up blood glucose levels.

Everywhere I looked I saw the infection that was going to send my blood glucose over the top, and like the bad guy in the Western, it was gunning for me. I was the cousin of the "clean freak," who runs a finger over every surface for dust; I was the "infection freak," checking my fingers for cuts, cringing at every sniffle. I was an obsessive-compulsive with the perfect tools for my trade—fear and an activity I could repeat again and again, testing my blood. From a slight cold to a hangnail, I became obsessed with testing my blood glucose—riddling my fingertips with tiny puncture wounds daily—for fear it might rise astronomically. It never did. I was stymied by the ordinary. I had a chronic condition that wasn't going anywhere, but I did not have a disaster on my hands. Time and familiarity with the situation eventually prodded me to get a grip.

The possibility of infection became only one more aspect of the fist of fate. This risk was simply more particular than others. Recently, I approached a severe bout of gastroenteritis with studied equanimity. I concentrated on drinking plenty of fluids and checked my blood glucose level only periodically. I did fine.

Hypochondria is normal. A little is fine, but a lot can start to hurt. My best advice is not to take on "the big picture" right away. Just take it one blood glucose reading at a time.

Now, when an unwitting acquaintance begins to quote the canon of complications that accompanies diabetes, I remind myself that this is a stereotype made possible because of the poor handling of an eminently manageable condition, and I remind the person that things don't have to be this way. "After all," I say, "look at me." My plan, of course, is to be perpetual proof of this statement—to live down the insensitive slings and arrows by being a continued, healthy contradiction. If this is my Sword of Damocles, I keep reminding myself that the blade is very dull, and I have somewhat more than a hair's breadth of control over whether or not it falls.

As I settled into a manageable degree of vigilance, I began to concentrate on a word—*endurance*. In order to do more than just survive—to live well—we need an ever-increasing measure of endurance. (I refuse to call it a mantra, but if it helps you to, go ahead.) Endurance is comprised of strength and patience. A person who possesses endurance automatically increases his or her reserve of all other inner resources. To develop endurance, we extend ourselves and overcome our natural resistance as it arises. It is physical work, but it is also intellectual and spiritual work. Endurance is both practical and mysterious, a physical and psychological phenomenon. It is composed of both stamina and drive. Ask any marathon runner, and their equation for what it takes to finish will be inexact—training, determination, and something else. Endurance is, among other things, the necessary underpinning for ambition itself. Concentrating on endurance gave shape to all the tedious elements of my routine. The details began to paint their own larger picture, which in turn increased my motivation and stamina for the program. These daily activities are training rituals in a marathon of self-care.

TELLING FRIENDS AND FAMILY

I know I'll sound like an "old fogy" (just imagine a crotchety voice), but I remember the train ride back to New York City on that snowy Friday just like it was yesterday. I love the snow, and so even my inevitable sorrow over what I perceived as my health crumbling at my feet lifted just a little. Snowflakes are one of life's great beauties.

As I stared out the window at the patterns the swirling snow created in the air, my thoughts were on my son. I found an impulse lurked to "protect him" from the news, old family detritus, the dead skin of growing up in a time when secrets loomed larger than life because they were kept from the children to protect them. Then I realized that when my parents divorced after all those secrets, I had been protected from nothing. It also occurred to me as a medical writer that my son would be dealing with health and health issues all of his life, and the more I could demystify the world of medicine and diffuse the issue of illness, the better prepared he would be to manage in the world. To make of the extraordinary, ordinary seemed key.

I'm not saying I was planning to stick his nose in my Glucometer. My plan was simply to be matter-of-fact. Oddly enough, or perhaps not so oddly, wanting to do right by my son steadied me. The plan worked. I sat on the couch in our tiny living room and showed my son, Dash, and his buddy, Teddy, my new machine. I can remember almost exactly what I said. "Dash, this is a test I have to do now to make sure there isn't too much sugar in my blood. I'm not sick. I just need to watch my blood sugar so that I don't get sick." I was direct. I was positive. Once you have children, you owe it to them not only to help them be happy, but to show them that you love life and can handle its adversities. After all, we give them the invitation to be born and enjoy the party; we better show them we enjoy it too.

I stuck to my one tried and true parenting concept (besides "give them love"); "tell them the truth, but don't tell them too much" and stopped there. I had made up my mind not to invite him to watch me stick my finger, not wanting to scar him for life any more than life forces us to. But he was curious about the Glucometer and wanted to watch. Not Teddy. Teddy was already in Dash's room watching *The Magic School Bus*. I won't say my son surprised me, but he did impress me. He kept assuring me it wouldn't hurt. "Don't worry mom, it'll just feel like a tiny prick." After all, he's had his finger stuck. He knows. I botched it the first time, but the second time I did just fine. My blood was 112 mg/dL, a number I will never forget, since it was already much improved from the day before. I was happy, and so was my son. And, I have to admit, it was probably a lot easier to prick my finger that first time with company. Now, almost two years later, I think I may have contributed to the makings of a physician. My son now helps. He feels my fingers to see which is "plump." He washes his hands so he can assist. (It's probably the only way I've ever gotten him to wash his hands voluntarily.) He even does the finger stick for me and waits for the numbers to come up. Believe me, I don't force this. And when he's bored—after all, Mom does this all the time—I don't expect him to sit and help. But there's something so dear and touching about this that I can only feel even better about having diabetes. I'm glad I told him, and I'm glad I wept on the phone to a friend the day before and not in his presence so that when I told him, I didn't feel the need to cry.

TELLING YOUR FRIENDS

I can keep anybody else's secrets, but I don't like having secrets of my own. If I were a spy, for example, I'd probably announce it. As I age, I'm not quite so blunt about confessing things, because I realize, for one thing, people just don't care that much. They're busy with their own lives and secrets.

As soon as I was diagnosed, I told my friends, and they gave me the boost of love and compassion I needed. I could cry and gain the strength I needed to be calm with my son. I told my mother, who helps out with my son. Much later, I told my father, whom I don't see very often. I told my dentist, my pedicurist, and my sometimes masseuse (who's also a friend). The more those who care for you physically know about your condition, the better your chances of protecting against infection and other problems.

As for others, I had enough poor responses from acquaintances (looks of near horror and then concern) that I decided to simply curb my tongue unless there was a reason to mention diabetes. Don't get me wrong; I don't hide it. (After all, I'm writing this book.) I've just learned the limits of honest compassion. I get what I need from my friends and then go on with my life. Oh, and by the way, I almost never tell waiters, unless I really like them. I simply say I'm allergic to carrots, which is only technically a lie.

IF YOU'RE DATING

What you say and when you say it will depend on how long you've been seeing whomever it is you're seeing. Obviously, if you have a close, committed relationship and he or she has a cell phone, you call from the doctor's office when you're diagnosed, if you feel like it. You've got nothing to hide, nothing to be embarrassed about, and you need to be close to those who love you at this time.

It's only other situations that may be tricky. For example, if you're going out on a blind date or a second date, moments or days after your diagnosis, what you say is going to depend on your personality type. If you're the kind that likes to test, doesn't want to waste time on a relationship that isn't going to go anywhere, and doesn't mind cutting to the chase, then by all means make your recent news a topic of conversation. If, on the other hand, you've spoken to friends, feel calm and in control, and would just like to have a pleasant evening, choose a movie instead of dinner out and just say you don't like popcorn. She or he will be impressed and ask no more.

The main thing is to feel comfortable with your choices. While you don't want to make a big deal out of your situation, your dietary restrictions, or anything else, you also don't want to be in a situation where the first time you prick your finger, he or she faints. This is the sort of person you may not want to spend much time with, much less the rest of your life.

SUPPORT GROUPS

Ask your doctor whether there is a support group for diabetes that he or she would recommend or whether there is simply another patient you might call just for support in getting you going. I don't attend an organized support group, but I'm in close phone contact with a couple of diabetics whom I love. I've also had a number of friends give my phone number to friends of theirs who are either newly diagnosed diabetics or not doing that well with their present treatment. I talk to them about my diet and recommend the diabetologists I think can help. I'm happy to report that each of these charges sent to me is doing better since they have embraced protein and found a diabetologist on the cutting edge of diabetes research and treatment.

In my travels as a diabetic, I've also discovered many acquaintances whose diabetes never came up until I had a diagnosis of my own. These include my lawyer, my accountant, a mother of two at my son's school who came to diabetes the same way I did (gestationally), a friend's brother, a friend's nephew. You name it. There are diabetics everywhere willing to chat with you about their ups and downs, good days and bad days. So I guess it must be true that there are nearly twenty million Americans who are diabetic. Isn't it comforting? You are not alone. If all these people can cope, you can too.

If you're an Internet aficionado, you might want to scroll through Web sites for information on diabetes support groups and chat rooms.

SOME ANNOYING SITUATIONS THAT MAY OCCUR

"Diabetes? Isn't that the one where you lose your feet?" My beloved-husband greeted me with this one. Since he hates to spend money, I replied, "Imagine how many taxis I'll have to take." If you don't want to be snide, you may want to heed Nancy Reagan's three immortal words: "Just say no." Or you could say that on the regimen you're following, you stand a good chance of outliving many non-diabetics—and all in one piece.

"Come on. One bite won't kill you." No, it probably won't, but that isn't really the issue. What you need your family and friends to understand is that your goals are long term. It's not a matter of life or death. It's a matter of keeping your blood glucose levels normal and consistent. If you don't do that, then it may become a matter of life or death. Before you indulge in that sweet dessert out of frustration or decide to shun old friends, give them a brief tour of the diabetic's pantry.

"But I cooked it myself." Never, never, never eat something out of guilt. This goes for non-diabetics as well as the rest of us, and it is one of the hardest lessons to learn, whether

our parents made us clean our plates or not. And never use guilt as an excuse to gorge. Many Americans are overweight due to this excuse. "Well, I had to finish it. He made it. He would have been insulted." Insults pass. Diabetes doesn't. The sooner you learn to give a polite refusal, the less chance there is of your wreaking havoc on your blood glucose levels every time you visit so-called friends. Remember, they mean well. But they don't know what you know. Until you fill them in, you can't blame them for wanting you to eat what they eat.

If you are with new friends and aren't comfortable going into detail about your food issues, you can also simply say, "No, thanks. I don't eat sweets." Remember, it's up to you to decide how much you want to tell anyone about yourself, and that includes whether or not you tell them you have diabetes.

3

Insulin: Hero of the Pancreas

Insulin is a wonder hormone, and once it was synthesized in the early twentieth century, it became a wonder drug. However, like all wonder drugs, insulin may be overprescribed and over-relied on by doctors who treat diabetes and by those who suffer from it. As with any wonder drug, insulin is not a cure. Almost all Type I diabetics would die without it, but if they do not take care of their overall health and if it is overprescribed, they may die with it, if not from it.

Knowing that you need to inject yourself with insulin is only the first step in getting the right treatment for your diabetes. Insulin is a naturally occurring hormone produced by the beta cells of the islets of Langerhans, which are in the pancreas. When you are producing insulin, the more glucose in the blood, the more insulin produced by the beta cells to process the glucose. Insulin is the saint, the general, and the teacher when it comes to the metabolization of glucose. It acts to regulate both the metabolism of glucose and the attendant processes that are necessary for the intermediate metabolism of carbohydrates, fats, and proteins. Insulin also promotes the entry of glucose into muscle cells and other tissues. It might be better to call insulin the wizard. Thus, when the wizard vanishes, due to the destruction of the beta cells that produce insulin, that magic trick of healthy digestion leading to normal blood glucose levels can no longer be performed.

In a health obsessed and disease obsessed culture, hormones, in general, still tend to get short shrift. In fact, except for estrogen and testosterone, hormones are heartily ignored, even with all the current hoopla about health and disease prevention. It makes sense that we would focus on the sex-related hormones, given that sex is a pet topic of this at once prim and provocative culture of ours. But without insulin and all of those other good hormones, we wouldn't even be able to worry about sex. If this were a political campaign, we might say, "It's the insulin stupid."

To dip into the mechanical for a moment: If the body were a car, the hormones would comprise the steering mechanism, which is absolutely vital to keeping the machine on course. These gems called hormones originate in the endocrine system, which is comprised of a number of glands. These glands include the pituitary, thyroid, and parathyroid glands in the head and neck, the adrenal glands and the pancreas in the abdominal area, and the ovaries or testes in the pelvic area. The endocrine system is a network that secretes hormones directly into the bloodstream to affect the function of specific target organs. They steer the body in the right direction every day, as long as everything is in working order.

Our hormone of choice, insulin, is produced in the pancreas by beta cells in the islets of Langerhans, as described earlier. As you know, insulin is secreted by the beta cells in response to glucose in the blood, glucose being the sugar that food is broken down into during digestion. Insulin then goes to work regulating the metabolism and also the attendant processes necessary for intermediary metabolism of fats, carbohydrates, and proteins. Insulin also promotes the transport and entry of glucose into the muscle cells and other tissues, thus delivering energy to the cells of the body. Insulin also regulates blood glucose levels in the process.

Think a little bit about how organic insulin—that which your body itself produces—works. When you eat a meal, insulin is released in direct proportion to how much is needed to regulate blood glucose at that moment. It stands to reason that if the job is a small one, the body does not release its big guns but provides only the right amount of insulin for the job. (We may not have a lot of common sense, but our bodies do.) This nicely regulated system has little to do with high-dose injections of insulin two or more times a day—the practiced method of insulin treatment, until the recent diabetes revolution finally began to gain some much needed momentum. Many diabetics have been injecting the insulin and then treating the medication with high doses of carbohydrates, which then have to be treated with more medication, thus setting another unneeded vicious cycle in motion. "Duh," you might say. (Or, as they say on *Saturday Night Live,* "What *were* you thinking?")

The simple answer is that whenever you add the word wonder to drug, you generally end up with a period of over-medication. In the case of insulin, for a long while doctors felt there was no choice. The patient would die without insulin; ergo, give him or her the insulin.

If you are an insulin-dependent diabetic and have been on insulin for years, discuss your insulin dosages with your doctor and see whether there is any room for adjustment. If your doctor is not willing to discuss re-evaluating your insulin needs, get a second opinion. If you have been newly diagnosed with diabetes, take the time to custom tailor your dosage requirements with your doctor, paying particularly close attention to blood glucose levels during the first month of treatment while you are fine tuning your dosage requirements. Among other extraordinary recent advances in how we are reorienting our approach to diabetes treatment, the mutability of insulin dosages is one of the most important breakthroughs. Rather than a rigid prescription that must not change, insulin therapy has become a mutable component in the treatment of diabetes. And it makes sense that as you age and your body and your needs change, your need for insulin should be re-evaluated as well. Nothing is static in this world, least of all the body's need for and use of a human hormone.

Never forget that the most important component of your treatment for diabetes should be that it is individualized, custom tailored to you and your needs. Just as no two diabetics are alike, no two treatment regimens for diabetes should be exactly alike. Your diet, your exercise strategies, and how you use insulin—or oral agents, for that matter—should reflect your individual needs.

INSULIN RESISTANCE

Put in the simplest of terms, insulin resistance is largely responsible for Type II diabetes. If you begin to overload your system with carbohydrates, your pancreas will respond by producing more insulin to cope with processing the carbohydrates. If you overload your system for years with carbs, your pancreas becomes stuck in an insulin overproduction mode. Concomitantly, your body becomes used to excessive amounts of insulin—you might even say inured—and more and more insulin becomes necessary to do the job of regulating blood glucose. Your cells become resistant to insulin. Whereas before the receptors on the cells needed only a small amount of insulin to keep blood sugar in the normal range, now they need more and more. The situation becomes chronic, and insulin resistance or hyperinsulinemia ensues. In much the same way as an alcoholic views liquor, your metabolism's relationship with insulin becomes one of too much is not enough. Eventually virtually all the insulin in the world can't handle regulating glucose. And voilà, the stage is set for Type II diabetes—the insulin you make is not equal to the task of keeping blood glucose levels normal. Call it the "all the tea in China syndrome." It's not the fault of the insulin; it's the resistance your body has built up over time. By the way, insulin resistance is usually accompanied by obesity, a predominant factor in the onset of Type II diabetes.

As you are developing insulin resistance, your blood sugar remains normal; the problem is occurring behind the scenes, as more and more insulin is required to do the same job. There is a test for hyperinsulinemia, but few doctors have it in their repertoire or use it, even when a patient is obese or has a history of diabetes in the family. The test measures your blood insulin level and can determine whether you have hyperinsulinemia. Since the test is rarely used, however, most people don't discover their insulin resistance until their blood glucose levels are elevated and they are diagnosed with diabetes.

Now, take the scenario in reverse. You follow this program and dramatically lower your consumption of carbohydrates. It's hard at first. You waver, but in staunch American pioneer fashion, you persevere. Stalwart in your resolve, you begin to notice a change. Your blood glucose levels are getting closer and closer to normal. By eliminating the mountain of carbohydrate, you begin to reverse the process of insulin resistance, slowly but surely. The receptors on the cells begin to be able to manage the job with less and less insulin. As this period of adjustment continues, the insulin you do produce becomes more efficient at doing its job. Put in nonmedical terms, it become "re-sensitized"—insulin resistance begins to "wear off." Eventually, insulin production normalizes, as do blood glucose levels. Low and behold, you've reversed insulin resistance—just another of the nearly miraculous effects of this new diabetes diet.

One of the benefits that accrues as insulin resistance diminishes is that managing blood glucose levels becomes easier. You should even find that over time your blood glucose levels fall even further into the normal range. This means that eventually you can increase the amount of complex carbohydrate in your diet—carefully and not dramatically—without a deleterious effect on your blood glucose levels. All of this good news should motivate you to start the program today.

IF YOU TAKE INSULIN

According to Dr. Richard K. Bernstein, almost all Type I diabetics—except those with the mildest cases, where the pancreas is still producing adequate insulin—should use rapid-acting insulin before each meal. On waking and at bedtime, long-acting insulin should be used to avoid blood sugar changes during the "fasting" period (when you are sleeping). This is in opposition to the now outdated but still often prescribed regimen of one or two very large doses of insulin taken during the day. This means that though you might have to inject yourself more frequently, you will actually be taking less insulin, and there is a far greater likelihood that you will normalize your blood sugar with the new regimen, as long as you follow the diet as well. If you are still on an old regimen, talk to your doctor about rethinking your insulin needs and read *Dr. Richard K. Bernstein's Diabetes Solution*.

Things are changing in the world of diabetes, and the news is all good. Finally, the goal is normal blood sugar for all. And in the case of diabetes, the end does justify the means. While insulin and oral hypoglycemic agents may have been overprescribed in the past, they are still partners in treatment—partners who have been relatively misunderstood until recently and can far better serve the health of the diabetic than they have. As a result, we are looking at a much broader horizon of individualized treatment plans for diabetics, and that is good news for both Type I and Type II diabetics. Even the distinction between

Type I and Type II may be becoming less important than focusing on the individual diabetic's needs. Call it a "rainbow coalition" of diabetics—the opening up of treatment issues for debate, the redrawing of treatment boundaries, and the redefining of the situation is good for all of us.

We Americans have an odd relationship with drugs that love/hate hardly describes. It's far more complicated than that. It's fairly safe to say that drugs in the United States are often overprescribed, and then, of course, the patient is told to quickly get off the prescribed drug before addiction—that naughty word of the '80s and '90s—takes hold. Then, of course, there are those who love our recreational drugs but would do just about anything to avoid going on medication to lower phenomenally high blood pressure—blood pressure that puts heart and health at risk.

In the case of "drugs" and diabetes, we're often talking about necessary medication. Though these medications have been overprescribed in the past, they should not be thrown out like that proverbial baby with the bath water. Insulin is not a drug; it's a hormone that has been manufactured to mimic the human hormone missing in a brittle diabetic's system. Oral hypoglycemic agents, which could be classified as drugs, are being refined so that they may be of the most use to the diabetic. In the past, almost every diabetic was medicated immediately. *This is not necessary and should not be the first approach. In many cases, diabetics have not even been given the chance to regulate blood sugar with diet and exercise. Now we can and must take that opportunity for ourselves first.* However, if the task proves impossible, insulin and oral agents—particularly metformin and troglitazone—can be lifesaving allies in the effort to normalize blood sugar. What holds true is that every diabetic, whether taking medication or not, must help manage normal blood sugar through diet and exercise. Drugs alone will not do this for you. So it's not either/or, it's what works for you.

Two good examples of the new ways in which insulin is being used can be seen in the treatment of Type II diabetics. Many Type II diabetics with poor control will end up doing damage to the pancreas and, therefore, the beta cells that produce insulin. Over time, such a diabetic will become insulin dependent (though a Type II diabetic) because virtually all beta cells will be destroyed, thus, for all intents and purposes, making the diabetic equivalent to a Type I. By using insulin before such damage occurs, the pancreas may be protected, thereby preventing complete insulin dependence. Insulin may also be used prophylactically in non-insulin dependent diabetics who become pregnant. By using insulin during your pregnancy, you can protect against pancreatic damage and possibly against becoming insulin dependent after your pregnancy. These are only two examples of a new phenomenon—creativity is finally being applied to diabetes treatment.

Oral Hypoglycemic Agents

You may try and try and still not be able to normalize your blood glucose levels with diet and exercise alone. If you can't, you can't. As we know, no two diabetics are alike, and the divining rod of treatment is this: Customize your treatment to your needs, and you'll solve the problem of diabetes. So if you can't do it alone, it's nothing to cry over. It's nothing to beat yourself up about. And please, don't blame yourself and don't look back. Look forward to getting the help you need, and look into oral agents so that you can be sure you have found the one that works best for you.

Of course, there are oral hypoglycemic agents, and there are oral hypoglycemic agents. All OHAs are not created equal. At present, the oral agents metformin hydrochloride and troglitazone offer the greatest benefits to patients. Troglitazone has just been made available and is expected to become the most popular oral agent of choice. Metformin is sold as Glucophage by the Bristol Meyers Squibb Company. What sets both metformin and troglitazone apart from other OHAs is that they both work by increasing the body's sensitivity to insulin, whether it is the insulin you produce or the insulin that you inject. This means that these OHAs serve a dual purpose. At the same time that

THE DAWN PHENOMENON

The dawn phenomenon or effect seems to be the exclusive property of insulin-dependent diabetics and occurs in most cases of insulin dependency. Dr. Peter Campbell and others from the Mayo Clinic fist documented surges of growth hormone early in the morning. Growth hormone is an insulin antagonist and is notorious for causing blood glucose levels to rise, sometimes a lot. Ergo, the dawn effect, a high blood glucose reading on rising or at least this was the thought way back then, a decade or so ago. Further research has shown that the dawn phenomenon begins approximately an hour before you awake and continues for 2 to 3 hours and that it results from the liver's rapid clearance of insulin from the bloodstream.

While the dawn phenomenon is basically the province of Type I diabetics, it's now clear that Type II diabetics may also be plagued by it. The rise usually continues after you've been out

they actively work to lower blood sugar, they also aid in developing the body's ability to use insulin. Thus, over time, they may aid the body in using insulin to lower blood glucose levels on its own, making lower doses of the OHA possible. Call them OHAs with a perk. Other OHAs include glyburide (DiaBeta or Micronase are trade names), chlorpropamide (Diabinese is the trade name), glipizide (Glucotrol is the trade name), and tolazamide (Tolinase is the trade name). These agents help to lower blood glucose levels, but they do not help to improve the effectiveness of the insulin you do produce. If you are taking one of these OHAs, discuss the reasons why with your doctor. There may be a particular reason that makes this OHA the right one for you. If this has simply been your doctor's OHA of choice, then discuss the possibility of switching to metformin or troglitazone with your doctor.

Generally OHAs are prescribed for Type II diabetics who cannot manage normal blood glucose through diet alone and/or who cannot manage to lose weight. The amount of the OHA and the timing of your doses are as important to your treatment as the type of OHA you take.

of bed for a while, wandering around the house waking up, but before you've eaten anything. How long it takes for blood sugar to rise and how much it rises depends on the individual.

The high reading is a problem that can be remedied fairly easily, with your insulin injection and breakfast. However, before the identification of the dawn effect, the first reading of the day—which was basically an inaccurate reading—was taken as the gold standard in terms of determining the amount of insulin you were to use throughout the day. A higher dose of insulin than necessary, in some cases a megadose, was being routinely prescribed for the patient.

Though the program outlined in this book will help insulin-dependent diabetics stabilize their blood sugars in the normal range, and with less insulin, the primary focus of the book is not insulin-dependent diabetes. I bring up the dawn effect as a particularly fine example of the recent advances in diabetes treatment. Until it was identified, in the mid-1980s, diabetics were routinely having insulin overprescribed. This meant they were eating more carbohydrates to "feed" the insulin than they had to and, in effect, contributing to the advancement of the disease they were trying to control.

Now insulin needs are calculated on daily blood glucose averages and with the help of the Hemoglobin A1C test, which calculates average bgls over a three-month period (see Glycolosylated Hemoglobin Measurement (HgbA1C)).

4

Preventing Prevention: How the Insurance Companies Encourage the Complications of Diabetes

Many of the policies of insurance coverage for diabetes are perfect examples of the time worthy saying "Penny wise, pound foolish." Preventive care for those at risk for diabetes and diabetics is often not covered by insurance, while the complications that cost the individual and the country hundreds of thousands and even millions of dollars are. And many of the costs in job hours lost, surgical procedures, and hospitalization could have been avoided had an early investment in prevention been supported by coverage.

Recently my present endocrinologist told me of a patient whose medical bills were hundreds of thousands of dollars a year, which the insurance company paid. (We assume not gladly.) Obviously, I said, he was not practicing "tight control," the term now used by those doctors in the know who are trying to help their patients normalize blood glucose levels and keep them there. My doctor responded that the patient had also been running high bgl levels for years before diagnosis, before he had even come to an endocrinologist for treatment. There you go.

This is the catch-22 of medical treatment and insurance coverage for diabetes: You can get what you need in terms of coverage if you are being hospitalized for ketoacidosis, insulin shock, or diabetic coma, or if you must have a partial limb amputation or eye surgery because of complications of diabetes, and yet you often cannot get reimbursed when you buy a Glucometer or equivalent home blood testing mechanism. Call it a cart of troubles without even allowing the horse to pull— call it what you will—but this backward thinking of the insurance industry tends to collaborate with ordinary human nature in preventing diabetics and pre-diabetics from getting the help they need before there is trouble.

Not only that, once diabetes results in complications, the drain on the financial system of the country is exacerbated by extended workdays lost and more medical costs. It makes no sense, and yet it continues. As they say on the street corner, "Go figure." But I guess nobody does figure. However, they should, because if you add it up, paying for every diabetic to have a Glucometer is an even better campaign slogan than "a chicken in every pot." And it's a terrific investment in the country's physical and economic health.

Now with President Clinton's 1997 endorsement of the commitment of funds to research on diabetes and the resultant increase in national attention to the subject, the insurance paradox may begin to change. Until then, remember that when it comes to diabetes, prevention *is* the cure. So even if you're paying out of pocket, your good health is worth it.

OVERHAULING THE STEREOTYPE

In June of 1997, diabetes made the front page of the *New York Times*. Bravo and brava! The news was salutary—new guidelines for testing, a national campaign to test all adults over the age of 45, and the endorsement of the Centers for Disease Control and the National Institute of Diabetes and Digestive and Kidney Diseases (see And What about the Future). Yet despite the extremely positive news and the upbeat tone, lurking further into the article was the same old "diabetes as death knell" stereotype. The first reference was phrased something like this: Scientists were worrying about the impact of telling "symptom free" diabetics that they have "a chronic disease with potentially devastating consequences" (*New York Times*, June 24, 1997). Well, here's one idea: Tell them that early intervention will protect millions of people from all of these "devastating consequences." Such guillotine rattling makes me want to say, "No, Chicken Little, the sky is not falling." Clearly, many Americans, from medical doctors on up and down the line, have yet to hear the message. A diabetic with consistently normal blood glucose levels has as good a chance as anyone of living healthily to a ripe old age. It's the diabetic who's not informed of his or her disease and not treated for the disease who begins to be at high risk for complications. Unfortunately, the stereotype is alive and well.

Diabetics have everything to live for, every chance of living well, and the chance of surviving their disease, never developing complications, and dying of something else entirely. And it is amazing that on the eve of the millennium, this disease is still perceived as anything from a nightmare you can't wake from to an incapacitating, debilitating, and unattractive problem that nobody really wants to hear about or talk about.

Diabetics who care for themselves well know a secret it may take the rest of the population longer to learn: The better we care for ourselves as we age, the greater enjoyment we'll get out of life and the easier the aging process will be on us both physically and mentally. Rather than being handicapped, diabetics may find themselves way ahead of the game.

We face the notion of aging with a grim determination. We want to do it well.

While saying "I'm diabetic, and I'm proud" may not get you front row seats at your favorite Broadway musical or get you into the hottest dance club in town, it sure beats hiding the fact or cringing when you say it. It might be time to start thinking of diabetics as individuals who are just slightly more aware of the risks of life on a daily basis—not as foreigners but as compatriots who got there, to the shores of mortality, a little bit sooner and have learned a great deal about how to appreciate life now, before it's too late.

It's up to each one of us to work to change the stereotype by controlling our condition and talking openly about the disease to others. By setting healthy examples, we'll begin to overhaul the ugly stereotype of the diabetic—albeit slowly. Recently, I heard a scare tactic ad for a local hospital that led off by saying that what diabetics fear most is the loss of a limb. Well, this is true, and it isn't true. And besides, people who are not diabetic also fear losing limbs. Who wouldn't? The difference is that with diabetes, nobody seems to want to start small. For example, when talking about cholesterol levels, one probably would not want to imply that every person with slightly elevated LDL cholesterol levels is bound to have a heart attack. But with diabetes, the tendency is to rush to injustice—first it's high blood glucose levels, then it's foot ulcers, then it's gangrene, and boom, you wind up at amputation. The other implication is that doom is inevitable and sacrosanct. Well, it's not.

There is a quiet revolution taking place in this country. You see it in the number of good, new books being published on diabetes. You see it in the innovative drugs now being tested (see And What about the Future). And it's happening among us—those who have been diagnosed with diabetes and are meeting the challenge of living well with the disease. While no one wants to glamorize a serious condition or disease, it's important to remember and to let the world know that life can be as joyful and productive and as healthy and creative after a diagnosis of diabetes as before. We now have the tools and the options to treat diabetes successfully and almost eliminate the risk of complications. The Glucometer, advances in research on diet and exercise, and advances in insulin production and the refinement of oral agents are helping to revolutionize how we treat and how we perceive diabetes.

All it takes is your commitment to self-care, and your life will begin to improve. If not in the palm of your hand, you have the secret to success at the tip of your finger. So go out there and fight the stereotype by being a living success story.

AND WHAT ABOUT THE FUTURE?

In changing how the world views diabetes, we are going to gain more and more support from the innovative research that is underway on new drug treatments and possible cures. The situation was never as hopeless as the common view of diabetes would have had you believe, but it has never been more hopeful. Not since the discovery of insulin have so many exciting research projects been garnering positive results.

It is generally agreed that even after 75 years of efforts to improve insulin therapy, the treatment is still imperfect, and most insulin dependent diabetics have trouble achieving optimal glucose control with insulin alone. Now, however, insulin analogs are being tested that may help make tight control easier for insulin dependent diabetics. Different types and combinations of insulin, different doses, and different timing of the doses are all part of current research projects.

In 1987, the hormone amylin was discovered by researchers at the University of Oxford. Amylin, like insulin, is produced by the beta cells. And like insulin, amylin levels normally increase after meals. Most interesting of all is that in diabetics, amylin response, like insulin response, is deficient. We now know that amylin affects at least two processes essential to normal glucose metabolism. First, it modulates the flow of glucose into the bloodstream from the gastrointestinal tract. Then it suppresses the secretion of glucagon, another pancreatic hormone, which stimulates the production of glucose by the liver. Since insulin acts to increase the outflow of glucose from the bloodstream to the tissues of the body, you might say amylin starts the job that insulin finishes.

A new drug called pramlintide is showing tremendous promise as a synthetic analog of human amylin. Pramlintide is in Phase III clinical trials in North America and has already been shown to be effective in improving glucose control in diabetics. You may wonder what's so great about that. After all, insulin does the same thing. Well, not only does pramlintide improve glucose control, but trials have shown that glucose lowering can be achieved through its use without an increase in hypoglycemic incidences, in direct contrast to intensive insulin therapy. The drug shows great promise for diabetes treatment in the coming years.

As recently as 1996, a U.S. study backed a study of implantable insulin devices, and the *Journal of the American Medical Association* reported that these devices can greatly improve diabetes treatment. Though external pumps have been available for over a decade, this one is quite different. It is fully implanted under the skin and injects insulin directly into the abdomen. The external pump injects insulin under the skin. The pump is about the size of a hockey puck; it is surgically inserted under the skin and then programmed to release insulin into the abdominal cavity.

A year-long study compared the pump with multiple, daily injections of insulin. Both methods were found to control blood sugar levels well, but patients using the pump had significantly fewer episodes of hypoglycemia (low blood sugar). This may be in part because the pump was also found to mimic natural production of insulin more closely. Other benefits included no weight gain. (The patients injecting insulin gained about 8 pounds.) Since many insulin dependent diabetics fear hypoglycemic reactions—which are uncomfortable and may include dizziness, confusion, agitation, sweating, and even fainting—they may tend to resist controlling blood sugar levels for fear they will go low enough to cause hypoglycemia. Thus, the pump may have the added benefit of aiding diabetics in aiming for tighter control of their blood sugar. The doctor refills a reservoir in the pump every 4 to 12 weeks, depending on the insulin demands of the patient.

Research is also currently underway on cloning beta cells. Once cells have been successfully replicated, they may then be transplanted back into the pancreas. This treatment depends on the existence of at least some beta cells in the pancreas; it cannot be used on brittle diabetics who produce no insulin and, therefore, have no beta cells. So far, the results are positive, and the cloning of beta cells is the best opportunity we have presently for a cure. This means you can essentially "cure yourself," as soon as the technique is perfected.

part 2

Tight Control Keeps the Doctor Away

Being a successful diabetic is not unlike being a successful slugger in baseball. It depends on the law of averages. One grand slam home run means nothing if you strike out the next hundred times at bat. But if you get on base with a single here and a double there, your average will reflect that you are a successful hitter. Of course, being a successful diabetic is harder. In baseball, the rule is three out of ten. Then your batting three hundred, a success by any standards. As a diabetic, you're striving for nothing less than blood glucose readings in the normal range every day. This section will help you bat a thousand, or at least close to it every day. The key will be to test your blood frequently at the beginning of your maintenance program so that you can keep blood glucose levels averaging in the normal range.

5

Me and My Glucometer

Electricity is considered the greatest of all inventions (after the wheel, I suppose). Just as electricity extended the day, so the Glucometer and other blood glucose measuring devices can extend the life span of almost every diabetic. After insulin, perhaps nothing has changed the life of a diabetic as much as being able to track blood glucose levels on a daily basis. Blood glucose measuring devices have done nothing less than revolutionize self-care for the diabetic.

If you don't have one, go to your local pharmacy and buy one now. Make sure the product you purchase gives accurate readings (some devices are more accurate than others). Few pharmacists are knowledgeable enough in this area to help you make an informed choice. So consult your doctor before you make your purchase. As with other technologies, advances are occurring so rapidly that you should probably "update" your blood measuring kit every 18 months to 2 years, just as you would your computer software. I use the "Glucometer Elite," which is manufactured by Bayer. (For simplicity's sake, therefore, I'm going to refer to my Glucometer, rather than to my blood measuring devices or outfits.)

If you shiver at the thought of pricking your finger, get over it. I did. Pricking your finger regularly may be the best thing that ever happened to you. There is no way you and your physician can work out the right treatment plan unless you keep a 24-hour record of the flux and flow of blood glucose levels.

I remember when my doctor first showed me how to use the Glucometer and told me to buy one. If not appalled, I was chagrined. The notion of sticking my finger and putting my blood on the test strip every day was just so clinical. It just seemed, well, so medical. Maybe it wasn't as bad as a shot in the arm, but it was bad enough. Now, I consider my blood Glucometer as one of my best inanimate friends. I see beauty and efficiency where I once saw only a lancet and a test strip.

Your physician needs a record of your daily "bloods" to develop your blood sugar profile and work with you to normalize those levels. There are several forms available for recording blood glucose levels. The best is probably the Glucograf, which was developed by Dr. Richard K. Bernstein; it can be ordered by telephone from Harrison Chemists at 1-800-829-1493. But if you can't stand the thought of yet another form to fill out (I know I couldn't), buy yourself a ninety-nine-cent notebook and keep your own diary. The important thing is the information. You'll need to record the time of day you tested, the activity (such as exercise or running errands) you were engaged in prior to testing, and whatever you ate at your most recent meal or snack. Think of it as scoring a ball game or solving a mystery. These are the clues you need to "crack the case" of normal blood glucose levels.

Whenever we have a new gadget, appliance, article of clothing, or any other new object or toy, we tend to become enamored, if not obsessed, with our new acquisition, in accord with human nature. This period of intense concentration lasts shorter or longer depending on the object and how much it was desired. You may say, "But nobody wants a Glucometer," and you would be right. I suppose it's more like a taste for olives, avocado, or caviar. It must be acquired. We wrinkle our noses at first, then we can't get enough. As medical divvies go, the Glucometer falls into this category. While at first it signifies illness, an unasked for life change, another responsibility, and another job to do, soon the Glucometer becomes a trusted pal, someone you can count on in the middle of a busy day. Then, once you begin to see the results of your new way of life, the Glucometer can become the bearer of good news. If you're having a bad day, a good blood glucose reading can make all the difference. And, like your shadow, or the late Jimmy Stewart's Harvey, the Glucometer becomes a trusted companion, good company, and positive reinforcement.

At the same time, you may also find that you become absorbed with the Glucometer and the blood glucose readings it can give you in a minute, any time, night or day. Like following the stock market, becoming mesmerized by the Internet, or becoming addicted to a cell phone, the Glucometer can take over. The first few weeks you may find yourself testing your blood far more frequently than your doctor recommended you do so. This is the courtship period, those rapturous times in which the world falls away, and it is only you and, in this case, a little machine that can't talk and only iterates numbers after imbibing a spot of your blood, so little, in fact, that Dracula would laugh. You may find the tips of your fingers riddled with pinpricks—enough to put old Sleeping Beauty to shame. I did. But this, too, shall pass—and should pass. (Just use a little vitamin E cream on your fingertips.) Otherwise, there would be a twelve-step program for Glucometer addiction and codependence, and there isn't. So, you're safe. In fact, I suggest you enjoy your little fling. Your absorption with your metal conscience can have a beneficial effect on your self-care, and it can be the beginning of a greater, personal understanding of your own blood sugar levels—testing your blood glucose levels often during the day can help you learn when your blood sugar does what and why. And since this disease varies so widely from person to person, it makes sense that the only way to treat it successfully is to become intimate with how your own blood glucose level reacts to what you do and what you eat during the day. I'm not going to say blood glucose levels are fickle. This would be insulting. But like the weather, they are changeable. Some diabetics find their blood sugar is higher in the morning. Some find it is higher after exercise. Whatever the idiosyncrasies of your own blood glucose, the more you know, the better equipped you'll be to make the changes needed to keep it in the normal range. It's probably not a good idea to start talking to your Glucometer too much, though a little one-way conversation now and then never hurt anyone.

When to Test Your Blood Glucose Level

If you are a Type I diabetic, testing your blood daily is of primary importance. How often you test it will depend on your insulin regimen and the plan you work out with your doctor. A rule of thumb is "the more often, the better," though within limits. In general, you should test your fasting blood as soon as you wake up, then test 5 hours after your injections of "regular" insulin. You should also test 2 hours after every meal and snack and before you go to bed. In addition, you should test your bgl before and after exercise or when you engage in more physical activity than usual (from shopping to sex or at any time when you feel your bgl might be higher or lower than you think it should be).

If you are a Type II diabetic who is just beginning this program, you should test your blood five times a day: upon rising, 2 hours after breakfast, lunch, and dinner, and before going to sleep. If things seem to be going smoothly, you can give up the mid-morning test. Then you should consult with your doctor and follow this regime once a week, as long as your doctor agrees. If you are just beginning your self-care for diabetes, you may want to test your blood daily for a week or two to help you custom tailor your regimen, to alert you if things are not going as you thought they were, and to give you vital encouragement when things are going well.

If you've had the flu or any infection or suspect for any reason that your blood sugar may be too high or too low, test your blood.

As time goes on, the relationship with the Glucometer waxes and wanes. Or mine did. Like some marriages I know, we were on again, off again. Now we've formed a lasting friendship, with only slight and even appropriate overtones of codependency. Once a week I devote a day to regular testing. This means four times a day—on rising, 2 hours after lunch, 2 hours after dinner, and before bedtime. Of course, if you eat late, you might as well call the third test a wash and just test at bedtime. If I exercise, I also test before and after exercise. Otherwise, I only test my blood when I'm sick with the flu or have an infection or am going through a stressful time, or—and this happens—when I simply become slightly paranoid.

TESTING YOUR BLOOD

There are many blood testing kits on the market. Some are better than others, so spend some time doing research before you make a purchase. They're not cheap, and they're often not covered by insurance.

I purchased a Glucometer Elite. It costs about $98 and comes in a handy-dandy, fake leather pouch/purse. Now, $98 may sound like a lot of money, and it is. But in most places where the Glucometer Elite is sold, you can get a coupon for a rebate of $40 or more rebate on your Glucometer (if you send it in with your receipt to the company), thereby cutting your cost almost in half. There are other choices. You need to make sure you purchase a product that gives accurate results and that you feel comfortable using. Remember, you'll be pricking your finger and placing your blood on a test strip, similar to a slide. You'll want to feel as comfortable with your apparatus as possible. While you can't pretest a Glucometer, you can discuss your choice with your doctor and with other diabetics you know.

Other equipment you will need on an ongoing basis include lancets (the better to stick your finger with) and test strips, upon which you will drip the blood evidence. You'll also want to keep a diary of your readings, so you'll need recording sheets or a diary. You will need a new test strip every time you test your blood. That's the most expensive part. While every doctor will tell you that you need to use a new lancet every time you test your blood, they'll also imply or whisper, under some table of discretion, that you don't have to change the lancet every time you draw your blood. I don't. Dr. Bernstein told me he doesn't. And I've never had a problem. The choice is up to you. As long as you are sure only you use the Glucometer, you are generally safe from infection. (I change my lancet about once a week, maybe less.) Before purchasing a Glucometer, check with your insurance company regarding what and how much they cover.

Just as there are many ways to skin a cat, there are many places to prick your finger. It is said that the dorsum is as good as the palmer when it comes to finger sticking. Let me explain. The dorsum is the back of the hand; the palmer is the palm. That's easy. You are supposed to get nice, juicy blood drawing areas on the dorsum. But if you are having a difficult time with control and need to check your blood often, you will want to consider the palm and the back of your hand because you will need new locations—places to stick that have not been stuck before. Palm up, palm down—you want to be able to avail yourself of a lot of locations. The more, the merrier is a way to protect yourself.

I, myself, however, never have found blood on the dorsum side. For me, it's a desert, but don't let that inhibit you from trying. I like the plump fingertips on the flip side of the nail. Call me old-fashioned; say I think too much about Sleeping Beauty. That's where I get my blood and get it easily. Once again, the only good program for controlling diabetes is one that is tailor-made for you. One mistake I made was pricking my left middle finger more frequently than any other. This became a habit partially because I'm right-handed and also because I seemed to get blood more readily from that finger. It started to hurt. I gave up my favoritism.

What Is the Amplitude?

Amplitude refers to the range or breadth of the vacillation in your blood glucose readings. To have a blood glucose reading of 95mg/dL at midday is a wonderful thing, if you're a diabetic. But if your blood glucose reading is 140mg/dL at dawn and almost as high as evening comes on, then your amplitude is too great. And when your amplitude runs amuck, you are in almost as much trouble as when your blood glucose readings are consistently high.

If you begin to control your blood sugar and you have an amplitude between 80 and 120, you shouldn't worry. The problem regarding amplitude begins when your fluctuations occur at high numbers. If your bgl is sometimes 120 mg/dL and then sky rockets to 200 or more (or if the reverse occurs and a hyperglycemic number drops to a hypoglycemic number with great speed), this is wearing for your pancreas and for your entire system.

Like love, blood sugar is never truly constant, whether you are diabetic or not. It is meant to fluctuate cyclically, depending on what you've eaten when and how long you've gone without food. But also like love, the extreme highs and lows are the most trying, and, like it or not, finding the middle range sustains us best.

Normalizing blood sugar and minimizing the amplitude can keep you a healthy diabetic. If you find you have normal blood sugars some of the time and then they spike and fall, discuss your treatment program with your doctor and consider medication, either in the form of oral hypoglycemic agents or small but frequent insulin doses or both. Amplitude run amok can be as dangerous as consistently high blood glucose levels.

Glucometers and most other blood testing apparatus that are spring activated and depend on finger-stick devices provide two covers for the lancet that pricks your finger. The Glucometer offers two choices. The clear or lighter colored cover is meant to be used if you have thin and/or sensitive skin. The gray or darker cover is meant for those with heartily callused, thick-skinned fingertips—fingertips like steel wool. The dark cover is thinner than the clear cover, allowing a deeper puncture by the lancet. You'll come to know how deep a puncture you need to draw the blood you need to obtain a reading. Try the lighter cover first. Obviously, the object is to make the minimum puncture to get the blood you need. You'll get better and better at this as you go along.

Now, here's how to use your trusty Glucometer. First, don't be afraid. It doesn't hurt, and you do get used to it.

- Wash your hands first, before you even get your test kit ready. Generally, if you haven't just been in the kitchen handling food, you really needn't worry. It's only food residues, such as a tiny drop of syrup from the waffles you just prepared for your family, that can cause erroneous but alarming high glucose readings. However, even though I'm rarely even near the honey pot, I do wash my hands prior to each test. Call me obsessive or paranoid about getting colds from shaking hands, it's still a good idea to wash your hands first, just in case. When you are waiting for the kids in the carpool lane, taking the train home from the office, hiking a trail that does not pass by a babbling brook, or for some other reason unable to get to a faucet and a bar of soap prior to finger sticking and blood testing, carry an individually wrapped Wash 'n' Dry with you. Though your doctor will probably swab your finger with alcohol prior to testing for blood glucose levels during your routine checkups, this is unnecessary to do at home. I've never used alcohol pads. I live with a 7-year-old boy who has many friends and many science experiments and a messy cat. I live with every manner of germ and natural disaster such circumstances imply and have not had so much as a red patch of skin after a finger stick, much less an infection. I swear by Dr. Bronner's peppermint soap and alternate this with a natural liquid soap that contains aloe vera to prevent dryness. The brand I use is called "Aloe Vera 80," by Natureade; it's available at most reasonably stocked health food stores. If, however, you find yourself uncomfortable with only a soapy washing between your finger and a needle prick, by all means swab with alcohol first. Remember, our goal is consistently normal blood sugars. However you get there, short of inhabiting a non-diabetic's body, is okay. The problem with swabbing excessively with alcohol is that it can dry your skin, which can cause you further problems as a diabetic.

- If you are testing your blood first thing in the morning, do a few finger exercises—flexing and straightening—to get your circulation going and warm up your hands. You'll find the blood will flow much more easily.
- Set up your test kit and test area. Open the foil wrapper that encases the individual test strip and place it by your Glucometer first so that you will not have to perform this task with a bleeding finger. Cock your pistol, that is, make sure your lancet is in place and ready to shoot.
- Prick a finger, any finger, and ready, set, go. Just as you try not to favor one child over another, try not to favor one finger over another. You are going to be doing this a lot. If you use the same finger over and over, you're likely to feel pain and cause bruising. Alternate fingers and hands, always. Think of yourself as a piano player. You need to use all fingers on your keyboard, which, in this case, is the lancet and the Glucometer.
- Once you have a large, visible drop of blood, place the blood in the appropriate area on the test strip. You'll know you've gotten enough blood on the test strip when the timer is activated. If the timer is not activated, remove the strip, tear open another foil packet, remove a new test strip, cock your Glucometer, and prick another finger. (You can use the same lancet. It's just you and your blood,

not somebody else's.) Depending on the system you are using, you'll have results within 1 or 2 minutes.

WHAT'S HYDROGEN PEROXIDE GOT TO DO WITH IT?

Though you'll spill very little blood pricking a finger, it can sometimes get on your clothing. I find that a quick wash with ice water usually takes the blood out nicely, but the application of a wee bit of hydrogen peroxide to the stain works best of all. I don't want to sound like Helpful Heloise for diabetics, but it does lift it right out. I've almost never spilled my blood anywhere but on my test strip, but once I did rush back to the keyboard rather too quickly and ended up with tiny spots of blood on E, D, and C, among others. I closed all files and used a Wash 'n' Dry on the keys. If you do find that your fingertip continues to bleed a bit, run it under cool water, then, using a Kleenex, apply pressure to the spot for a moment or two, and it will stop.

Glycolosylated Hemoglobin Measurement (HgbA1C)

If you test your blood glucose levels every day religiously, there is probably little the hemoglobin A1C test will tell you that you don't already know. But it is invaluable for anyone who is not quite so religious and still important even for those of us who keep a daily record—if nothing else, it proves to the doctor that we're telling the truth.

The hemoglobin A1C tests your bgls for the last 2 to 3 months. Not very long ago, this test required that blood be drawn. But now, wonder of wonders, it can be done with a mere fingerstick, just like your daily tests with the Glucometer. (At my last visit to my endocrinologist, I had the results in minutes—or as long as it took the nurse to run the test, talk to other patients, answer phone calls, and finally get back to me.) I was very excited. My blood glucose was in the normal range of normal—good news. The caveat with this test is that it may either register numbers higher or lower than the true numbers. If you are testing your blood regularly and keeping track of the results, this should not be of great concern, since you have something to test the test against.

Hemoglobin A1C is normally a tiny part of your total hemoglobin supply. However, if your blood glucose levels have been elevated, glucose will stick to the hemoglobin A. (Normal hemoglobin A accounts for

LET YOUR BLOOD GLUCOSE BE YOUR PILOT

Evidently when asked on her deathbed, "What is the answer?" Gertrude Stein responded, "What is the question?" If you're not feeling there's is a whole lot to be grateful for in the diabetes rag, you can be thankful that in the case of diabetes, as complex a condition as it may be, the question is simple— "What is your blood glucose level?" If your answer is "Well within the normal range," then you've hit the jackpot. When people say things like, "Oh, you're a diabetic? How ___," (scary, hard, terrible—you pick), they only know the beginning of the story. The end of the story is that as long as you keep your blood sugars regulated, you won't suffer the effects of diabetes. Once you start to work your blood sugar levels as careful and energetically as a good comic works the room, you become privy to one of the great medical sleights of hand of all time— you know . . . the magic that will make diabetes "disappear."

about 97.5 percent of your red blood cells.) When blood glucose l evels are consistently high, red blood cells become altered over time and a compound called glycolosylated hemoglobin forms. When blood glucose levels are normal or close to normal, a small percentage of hemoglobin becomes glycolosylated. When diabetes is poorly controlled, however, the level of glycolosylated hemoglobin is much higher and can be as high as 12 percent. Such a reading indicates that blood glucose levels have been consistently elevated for a period of a month to 6 weeks. Normal readings indicate normal blood glucose levels for the same period.

Once glucose attaches itself to hemoglobin A, it will remain there for the life span of the hemoglobin A cells, approximately 120 days. Therefore by measuring the A1C, your doctor is recording an accurate record of your blood sugar activity over a matter of months. Like a summary report or term paper, it's a great way to keep track of how you're doing.

My doctor gives me this test every time I visit, which used to be every 3 months and is now every 6 months. If you are not receiving a hemoglobin A1C test regularly, ask your doctor why and ask for one.

Once you begin to realize how straightforward the essence of the disease is, you can begin to focus your energies on maintaining normal blood glucose levels throughout the day, minimizing fluctuation and making corrections as quickly as possible.

To go back to the mystery analogy, you are the detective, and your blood glucose levels are your clues. If you had fresh fruit for breakfast with a slice of whole grain bread, and you test your bgl and it's high, you need to rethink breakfast. If you have been rigidly restricting your intake of all carbohydrates and decide to try a meal that includes a lentil salad and a half slice of whole grain bread, try testing your blood glucose level 2 hours later. If it is within the normal range, perhaps it is time to try adding more complex carbohydrates to your diet.

Your blood glucose levels will help you chart your daily course and mark your path toward better overall health and nutrition. If mysteries don't work for you, think of your blood testing kit as the rudder that keeps you on course. Never be without it.

6

Stress and Your Blood Glucose Levels

By now it's common knowledge that stress can affect our health, but except for the "knee-jerk" reaction between intense stress and a rise in blood pressure, the connection is more mysterious than not. A friend who seems to live a highly stressed life may never get sick, and your calmest friend may be often ill. It seems, then, that stress is not in the eye of the beholder but in the body and personality of the individual.

Does that stress directly affect blood glucose levels? Over the long term, probably not, or I would hardly be able to manage my bgls as well as I do. I lead a highly pressured life. I don't lead it in the fast lane, but believe me there's pressure from all sides. And where there's pressure, there's stress, the kind that could make Atlas shrug. And still, I keep my blood sugar in normal range. It's something to hold onto I guess, a talisman. Something to pat myself on the back about when all else is in chaotic shambles. It's the one thing in my life that doesn't seem to be held together with glue, tape, and paper clips.

Having said all that, however, no one can tell me stress didn't have something to do with pushing my glucose levels over the edge. Perhaps the stress, per se, did not contribute to the actual diagnosis, but how I was living because of the stress did. I ate as well as I could and tried to keep exercising, but the pressures were enormous, time and money were tight, and the first thing that always got crossed off the list of things to do was "take care of myself." I played fast and loose with meals, embraced wine in the evening a little too heartily, went hungry when I was busy, and, all in all, slowly but surely wore myself down. Whatever you believe about stress and the immune system, I know that year cut into my body's resources to defend itself against intruding viruses and everything else that comes along to threaten our health. I got more colds. I even got the flu. And my hide is as tough as an elephant's when it comes to resisting the flu. I was a prime candidate for disease to infiltrate, and then it did.

So does stress affect blood sugar? The answer is no, and the answer is yes. Certainly, if you are in a crisis period and you neglect to take care of yourself, there may be consequences to your health. It is a good idea to do an inventory of your self-care habits, whenever megabytes of stress enter your life, just to make certain you are not being neglectful and allowing openings for any manner of health problems.

There is one time, however, when stress can have a direct effect on blood glucose levels. That's when you experience short-term, high-volume stress, which then causes the release of adrenaline. This can trigger a rapid rise in blood sugar. This occurs because the adrenaline surge triggers the release of a counter-regulatory hormone called epinephrine. Epinephrine, in turn, triggers the liver to begin to convert its store of glycogen to glucose, and voilà, up goes your bgl. The same phenomenon occurs during aerobic exercise, which also causes an adrenaline surge (see Part V, The Sisyphus Strategy: Lift Weights, Walk Uphill, Don't Stop). If you are a Type II diabetic who still produces plenty of insulin, this rise is usually corrected naturally and quickly. If you are a Type I diabetic and you experience periods of acute stress in your life, you should test your blood glucose level after such periods. If it is elevated, you should discuss the situation with your endocrinologist. You may want to work out a system whereby you adjust your blood sugar with a small "emergency" amount of insulin so that your blood sugar level does not remain elevated for a long period of time.

Stress may not have a direct correlation to a rise in blood glucose levels, but stress definitely affects your overall health and your eating habits. If you are under a great deal of stress, you may begin to use food to comfort or relax you, which may cause you to start making the wrong choices for the health of your blood. So if you are experiencing prolonged periods of stress and seem unable to remain committed to keeping your blood glucose levels normal, talk to your doctor. You may want to consider seeing a therapist to discuss the issues that are causing you stress. In some cases, your doctor and therapist may recommend medication, such as an antianxiety drug or an antidepressant, for a period of time. These drugs will not raise your bgl and, in some cases, may lower it.

There are also things you can do to control the level of stress in your daily life. Here is a short list of possible stress busters:

- Walking (see A Meditation on Walking)
- Doing breathing exercises (see Don't Forget to Breathe)
- Listening to music
- Taking up a hobby
- Exercising
- Meditating
- Practicing yoga (I have only my personal evidence, but I do find that my blood sugar is routinely a few points lower about an hour after my yoga class. But it's good enough for me.)
- Relaxing (ha, ha—but try anyway)
- Getting a good night's sleep

If you experience any major life changes or crises, your stress level is bound to rise; this means that your blood glucose levels may rise too. If and when any major changes occur in your life—from losing a spouse, to losing a job, to the commencement of menopause—pay particular attention to your blood glucose levels, testing more frequently, and contact your doctor if they begin to be elevated. In fact, you should contact your doctor in any case and enlist his or her support in managing your diabetes during this difficult time. Some universally recognized crisis points are:

- The death of a child
- The death of a spouse
- The death of a parent
- Divorce
- Caring for a critically ill child
- Menopause
- Losing a job
- Moving
- Retiring
- Caring for an elderly parent

Don't Forget to Breathe

You'd think breathing would be easy. You'd think breathing would come naturally. But studies show that we don't breathe deeply enough. So don't forget to breathe deeply.

OVERCOMING YOUR RESISTANCE

One of the hardest parts of being diagnosed with diabetes comes at the moment when your doctor begins to tell you what to do—not ask you, tell you. Suddenly, you are back there, sitting in front of whatever figure of authority it was that first gave the word *rebellion* meaning for you, and guess what you want to do? You rebel. Whatever your form of rebellion may be—junk food, hot dogs on white rolls, sweets, or Margaritas—suddenly you want to mainline. The idea that somebody is telling you that you can't indulge makes it that much harder for you not to.

This is the period in which you have to battle your own inner demons. And, like all great quests in life, wrestling what's inside you will be equally as hard as wrestling any real enemies. And notwithstanding the importance of cutting-edge medical care and a few lucky breaks, how you manage your own resistance is the linchpin of your treatment, the compass that will chart your course. Nothing is more important.

If you find yourself bridling when faced with another omelet, and longing for pizza, you need to rethink your orientation. You're probably thinking something like "I can't do this my whole life, so why even try?" or "Nobody's going to tell me what to eat. My life is hard enough. This is one of my few pleasures. So, full speed ahead, forget the consequences." As the experts would tell you, you're acting out.

Think again. The first step is to forgive yourself. Every good diabetic ends up where you are, sooner or later—up against the wall and banging your head, and the wall is inside you. This is the moment of recognition—the "I am my own worst enemy" moment without which it would not be life. Once you've realized such a crisis is inevitable, all you have to do is find a way to deal with the crisis successfully.

This involves looking at things from another angle. What you are embarking on is not a diet or a repressive regime. If you look at it that way, you are sure to fail. You're not facing a paucity of flavors or an austerity budget of gustatory pleasures you're making a conscious choice to change your life. This is an opportunity, not a life sentence.

Think of yourself as the conductor. Your organs, hormones, and blood comprise your orchestra. Through collaboration and direction, you make music. Without such teamwork, all you get is noise. When you start collaborating with yourself, you move from the dissonance and friction of resistance to harmony.

Finally, do your best not to become bored. Boredom is the handmaiden of self-defeating, if not self-destructive, behavior. Vary your meal plan and vary your exercise plan—before you become bored (unless you are one of those that thrives on routine). Go to the movies; take walks. As they say, get out of your head.

7

Sex, Diabetes, and Rock 'n' Roll

I'm not going to say that life begins when you're diagnosed with diabetes, but if you make the investment you need to make to manage your condition well, life may be even better than it was.

A SATISFYING SEX LIFE

Let's face it. One of the first questions, whether voiced or not, that everyone has when a life-changing circumstance occurs is usually "How will it affect my sex life?" In the case of diabetes, there are many answers. The good news is that there are more positive answers than negative ones. Your condition may not affect your sex life at all. In fact, your sex life may improve as you lose weight, get in shape, and start eating a healthier diet. The bad news is that if you are not diagnosed early and you already suffer from some diabetic complications, particularly neuropathy, sex, in particular for men, may be affected.

THE RISK OF IMPOTENCE

Unfortunately, a certain number of diabetic men do develop sexual problems, including sexual dysfunction, by middle life. Impotence caused by diabetes is most often caused by neuropathy (nerve damage, in this case, caused by diabetes), one of the most common complications of the disease when tight control has not been maintained over a long period of time.

Even though not enough studies have been done to directly relate impotence and other sexual problems to the severity of the diabetes, the general wisdom is that, in fact, sexual problems in male diabetics are related to poor blood sugar control over a number of years. In other words, it's progressive. And once again, controlling your blood glucose levels can solve your problems. If nothing yet has motivated you to take seriously just how important consistently normal bgls are to your health and well-being, maybe protecting your sex life will.

Impotence is not, however, a direct corollary of diabetes. In fact, many men who have been diabetic for 50 years and not exercised perfect or tight control have active sexual lives and do not suffer at all from impotence. It's simply that the risk is there, and the tighter the control you keep, the lower your risk will be.

When it is the result of diabetes, impotence never develops suddenly, but always gradually. If you find you are experiencing episodes of impotence, talk to your doctor immediately. He or she will probably suggest that you be examined by both a urologist and a neurologist. If there are no obvious physical factors contributing to your diabetes, you may be advised to undergo what is called an NPT evaluation. NPT refers to nocturnal penal tumescence. This will involve some time, some sleeplessness, and probably some embarrassment, but remember it's for a good cause. All sexually functional men experience periodic, nocturnal erections while they are sleeping. Monitoring these erections, then, is the infallible test to see if your impotence is caused by physiological or psychological reasons. If you do experience erections at regular intervals, your impotence is most definitely not caused by physiological problems, and this good news has cost you no more than one rocky night's sleep in the sleep disorders clinic of your local hospital. If you do not experience regular erections during sleep, then your problems are physiological, and at least you can now begin to isolate what the problem is and solve it.

Whatever you do, don't suffer in silence. Get help, because there is help.

DIAGNOSIS AND TREATMENT OF IMPOTENCE

If poor control of your blood glucose levels is causing your impotence and you still have trouble managing tighter control, you should seek your doctor's help. He or she may suggest you work with a nutritionist and may work with you to maintain tighter control through using insulin or oral agents. If you are already using insulin, the amount you are using and the frequency with which your are injecting insulin may need to be re-evaluated.

If your impotence is caused by neuropathy, there are options. Your doctor may suggest that you try a drug called mytelase. Mytelase has proven effective for some men in increasing the function of nerve endings and therefore the sensitivity of the penis. Unfortunately, mytelase sometimes causes violent cramping, a very painful side effect that then calls for an immediate dose of atropine to counteract the cramping. The good news is that new drugs are now being tested that can also increase the functioning of nerve endings and, thus, effectively treat the underlying neuropathy that is causing the impotence.

One other option is a penile implant. While this is hardly something any man thinks of without a shudder first, major strides have been made in designing penile implants that are comfortable and that allow satisfying sexual intercourse, including orgasm and ejaculation. There are now three types of penile implants: one you pump up, one that is semirigid, and one that is rigid all the time—a fantasy perhaps of many men, but not something, I imagine, they really want.

A more complicated, inflatable device is also available. Usually referred to as an inflatable erectile prosthesis, this device operates by allowing the simulation of an erection by inflation and deflation by command. If you are considering any type of penile implant, you should discuss the pros and cons with your doctor as bluntly and thoroughly as possible before taking such a step. Obviously, your partner should also share in the decision making process with you, and, in addition, you may want to seek counseling or therapeutic help.

Obviously, or not so obviously, solving the issue of your impotence through the breathtaking miracles of technology should not lessen your motivation to exert tighter control over your blood sugar. You may have solved one problem, but the underlying condition, your diabetes, must still be handled, which means managing it well. Sex enhances life greatly. However, if you are in poor health because blood glucose levels are raging, even sex isn't going to make you feel all that much better. Only taking care of your health will. So, once again, you are and must be the master of your condition.

Now, Viagra has arrived on the scene and changed many men's and many couple's lives. While there have been no clinical studies directly involving diabetic men, so far the risk factors appear to be the same as those for other men. In other words, if you have a heart condition or other complications related to diabetes, you are probably not a candidate for Viagra. However, if you are in generally good health, but have problems with impotence you might be a candidate. Discuss this with your doctor. In general, if you already have complications arising from diabetes, Viagra may not be the right solution to your problem. Never fear, as this book is being written, much progress is being made in terms of effective, healthy ways to deal with impotence.

FERTILITY

Unless neuropathy and resultant impotence are present, diabetes does not affect a man's fertility. If neuropathy has already occurred, a condition known as "retrograde ejaculation" may preclude insemination. When the nerve impulses to the penis are impaired and ejaculation occurs, the semen, which includes the sperm, may be unable to flow because the circular band of muscle fibers (the sphincter) will not open. The semen then flows back into the bladder. In this situation, intercourse, including orgasm, may not be at all affected, but insemination is obviously impossible.

CONTRACEPTION

While diabetic women seem to be free of any complications that impede the enjoyment of sex, the contraception they choose can affect their health. The barrier methods, the condom or the diaphragm, are the safest methods of contraception for the diabetic woman. If your mate or spouse is reluctant to use condoms, remind him that he is out of touch with the latest styles in contraception and its first cousin, safe sex. Condoms are all the rage now. If you don't use one, it's questionable whether you've actually had sex at all.

If, however, barrier methods do not appeal, you should avoid using the "pill," the most prescribed form of oral contraception. According to recent studies, a progestogen-only oral contraception has been found to have the fewest side effects for diabetic women. The major side effect is irregular menstrual periods. The classic oral contraceptive, the "pill," does not have such an innocent track record with diabetic women. Studies have shown that your glucose tolerance may be lowered by the hormones in the pill—not a good thing. In addition, this increased lack of tolerance may then trigger your existing insulin supply to become even less effective. Finally, there are also the general risks associated with the pill—an increased risk of blood clots and cardiovascular disease and an increased risk of vaginal infections. Since one of your goals is to minimize the number of infections you acquire, this is one more reason to avoid the pill.

The IUD (intrauterine device) is also not recommended for diabetic women. IUDs are associated with an increased risk of vaginal infection, just what the diabetic doesn't need. In addition, oddly enough, studies have shown there is a higher failure rate among diabetic women using IUDs than among the general public. This may be due to an altered metabolic reaction of the uterine lining (endometrium) because of the device. Whatever the reason, stay away from the IUD.

If you've already had your children, you and your partner may want to consider sterilization, which means a vasectomy for men or a tubal ligation for women. The vasectomy is a simpler, safer, less expensive procedure, and the risk of possible complications with a vasectomy is lower.

Norplant and Depoprovara are now available as alternative forms of birth control for women. Depoprovara can be injected every three months, avoiding the daily usage of contraceptives. Norplant is inserted under the skin. Both forms of birth control have been associated with a number of side effects, such as moodiness, jitters, and sweats. Both of these have the same risk of side effects for diabetic women as they do for other women. At the time of the writing of this book, a great deal of research on safer, more effective forms of birth control is underway.

SEX AND AGING: IT'S NOT JUST ABOUT DIABETES

For most of us, being diagnosed with Type II diabetes coincides with the inescapable aging process. And in the area of sexuality, the effects of the newly diagnosed condition and the ongoing process may overlap and/or be confused. First and foremost, as we age, we all get a little bit slower at one thing or another naturally. This may be particularly true in the case of an erection. A man may want sex just as much and be just as excited as he was when he was 25, but it may take longer for the evidence to show. This natural slowing down should by no means be confused with incipient diabetes-related impotence. If you or your partner start to think this way, it could have debilitating, psychological effects, and the situation will only get worse. When it comes to sex, what really changes in the middle and later years has to do with time and certainly not quality.

What men will notice first is probably that getting an erection takes longer, and once you have an erection, it may not be as hard as in your younger years. They may also find that it takes more direct stimulation to obtain an erection and reach orgasm. The time it takes to reach orgasm is also longer, and the ejaculation may not be as powerful. Such changes make many men feel that they are under even greater pressure to perform.

What women may notice is that they do not lubricate as quickly. Their labia may not become engorged and breasts may not swell up as much. Also, the nipples may not become as hard. The most common complaint among women has to do with lubrication taking longer and often being inadequate.

Such changes in men and women as they age are normal and to be expected. They should not be confused with complications of diabetes or be blamed on your diabetes. We and our non-diabetic brethren all get to experience such iffy joys of aging together.

In most cases, when you are managing your diabetes well, feeling better, and losing weight, you'll find your sex life improving along with the rest of your life. As you lose weight, you'll also start to feel more desirable, another plus when it comes to the libido and its often confounding nature. So, unless the complications associated with your diabetes are severe, you will probably find you're in better shape sexually than you were before.

OF INSULIN PUMPS AND SEX

Some insulin dependent diabetics can regulate blood sugar more effectively if they wear a pump. Pump designs are becoming more and more streamlined so that in many cases wearing a pump need not interfere with your sex life at all. If, however, you find that your pump interferes with finding a comfortable position or otherwise impedes your enjoyment, discuss removing your pump for the duration of sexual activity with your doctor. In most cases, your doctor will approve. Just remember, in the afterglow, to put the pump back on.

SAFE SEX: ONE LAST WORD

Sure, you know this. You've been bombarded with it by now. But once again, if you're dating someone new, you must take precautions. This means using condoms all the time. Nothing else will do, and nothing could be worse for you than any kind of venereal infection, mild or wild. You don't want to send your blood sugar through the roof just for a roll in the hay. So practice what I preach.

DIABETES, DRUGS, AND ROCK 'N' ROLL

If you like rock 'n' roll, it's good for you, which makes it good for your diabetes. Drugs and diabetes, on the other hand, deserve a certain amount of discussion. In some cases, a prescribed drug you may be taking for another condition may have a negative effect on the management of your blood sugar. Make your doctor aware of any prescribed drugs, any over-the-counter medications, any homeopathic or herbal remedies, and/or any recreational drugs you may be taking. From a simple decongestant to your blood pressure medication, the drugs you take can affect your blood sugar and make controlling your diabetes more difficult. In particular, it should be noted that taking diuretics can inhibit the release of insulin. So cross all diuretics off your list.

Now, about so-called recreational drugs.

MARIJUANA

Though marijuana is now being touted not only for its pleasurable effects but also as having some medicinal value, this is not so for the diabetic. Getting "stoned" can mask insulin reactions and may also make you unaware of when you need to eat. You may let mealtime pass by because you are enjoying yourself, or if you are one of those people who react to dope with a case of the grand munchies, you may be tempted to munch on foods that are downright bad for you.

AMPHETAMINES AND NARCOTICS

Amphetamines are stimulants and may affect your blood sugar in unexpected ways—either by raising or lowering it rapidly. Narcotics, such as cocaine and heroin, can alter how you absorb sugar and in this way affect your blood sugar levels. Obviously, you should steer clear of these drugs for many health reasons. Just add protecting your newly regulated blood sugar to the list.

ANTIDEPRESSANTS

Antidepressants may be the one exception to the rule when it comes to drugs and blood sugar. Diabetologists I have consulted say antidepressants may even have a beneficial effect on blood sugar, since they tend to lower anxiety and relieve stress. If you are on an antidepressant or considering taking one, discuss the drug with your doctor.

A NOTE ON GINSENG

Ginseng has recently been lauded as an alternative medicinal cure-all for almost anything that ails you. Not so for the diabetic. The steriod-like effect associated with ginseng can raise blood sugar.

TOBACCO

Smoking kills everyone, but it can kill a diabetic sooner. If you smoke, you must quit now. This has been said many ways, many times, probably by your doctor, your spouse or partner, your children, your mother, your father, your friends, maybe even your boss, and certainly the message has bombarded you from every conceivable media source (except, of course, those billboards that still advertise cigarette brands). Perhaps you rationalized, "Well, it won't kill me now." But you can't do that anymore. Every cigarette you smoke adds to your risk of complications from diabetes. So the truth is, you have to stop now. If you can't, get help from your doctor; discuss with him or her the "patch" and a nicotine substitute gum. You may also find a support group helpful. If you do nothing else to help manage your diabetes with self-care, at least give up smoking.

Tobacco Truth

Cigarettes kill over 434,000 people every year, according to the EPA (Environmental Protection Agency). And the EPA has now listed second-hand smoke as a group A carcinogen, along with asbestos and benzene. There are nearly four thousand chemicals in cigarette smoke, at least fifty of which are known cancer-causing agents. Among these chemicals are lead, arsenic, ammonia, nicotine, benzene, vinyl chloride (used in the production of plastic), and cadmium (used to make batteries). In addition, somewhere between 2 and 6 percent of cigarette smoke is carbon monoxide, a toxic gas often used in larger doses as a means of committing suicide.

THE LIFE OF THE PARTY

As the great poet Ranier Maria Rilke said, "The point is to live everything . . ." He was writing to a young poet who had many questions about art and about life—those two biggies. The mature poet's advice was to live even the questions, since it is through experiencing the questions that we may discover the answers. You might say managing diabetes is a journey within the larger journey or quest, and on that journey, the point for the diabetic is to live everything, but without unnecessarily jeopardizing the delicate balance of your continued good health. There will be some compromises you may have to make for this to happen. They may be as simple as carrying a little plastic bag filled with almonds with you wherever you go or as complicated as packing your insulin in airtight plastic bags when you go on that safari you've always dreamed of. What is equally important to the delicate balance of your emotional acceptance of your condition is that you are willing to make these compromises without seeing them as a sacrifice. Giving is good, and generosity—from generosity of the spirit to being generous with love, good works, or even cold hard cash and time—is a true act of grace. But sacrifice, unless you're applying for sainthood (and even then it's dubious), is not good for us. Sacrifice leads to resentment, and resentment leads to rebellion. And in this case the only person you have to rebel against is yourself, which will only jeopardize your health.

A truth about living well with diabetes is that maintaining your quality of life is equally as important as maintaining good control over your blood glucose levels. The old saying "the two go hand in hand" was never more true than in this case. When you are emotionally content, you are far more likely to take care of yourself, and taking care of yourself, in turn, will make you feel better and add to your sense of well-being and contentment. So, go to the party. Have a glass of wine and dance all or half the night (depending on how much you need your sleep). Just don't drink the spiked fruit punch and don't eat the eclairs.

And remember to count your blessings. If the list is short, count them again.

8

Pregnancy and Diabetes

In most cases, when diabetes is well controlled, a healthy pregnancy is possible for both mother and fetus. Only a decade ago, a diabetic woman might have had trouble conceiving and had a high risk of losing the baby and of jeopardizing her own health. That all of this has changed so quickly is one major indication of how much real progress is being made in treating diabetes and preventing complications.

It is never more important to plan ahead for pregnancy than it is if you are diabetic. Planning ahead can make the difference between a smooth pregnancy with a healthy outcome for mother and child and a pregnancy with problems. If you are considering getting pregnant, first and foremost you'll want to exert even tighter control of your blood glucose levels. The steadier your bgls are going into your pregnancy, the better your chances are for it to be normal and healthy. Then your goal during pregnancy is to keep your blood glucose levels as consistently normal as possible.

As long as your diabetes is under control when you conceive and you work closely with your gynecologist, specialist, and other members of your medical team to keep tight control of your blood glucose levels during the pregnancy, you can look forward to a positive outcome. You will, however, probably be scheduled for a C-section delivery. This is par for the course for diabetic women, including those with gestational diabetes only, for two reasons: concern over the safety of the mother's health during delivery and concern with the birth weight of the baby. The most common effect of the mother's diabetes on the baby is a high birth weight. This usually only occurs when blood glucose levels have fluctuated or been routinely higher than normal. Still, even if you have maintained tight control, you will probably be scheduled for a C-section.

PLANNING AHEAD

Planning ahead for the diabetic should include the same elements as for a non-diabetic, such as eating a healthy diet and exercising so that you are in good shape. You should also make every effort to arrange your life in such a way that you have more leeway to take it easy in case you are tired or suffer from morning sickness during the first trimester. Later on, you may simply want to take a little more time to enjoy life before your wonderful and time-consuming baby turns it upside down. Your pre-pregnancy plan should also include some other components particular to your needs as a diabetic. Before you try to conceive, the following elements of your pregnancy plan should be in place:

- Your diabetes should be under control with blood glucose levels consistently normal.
- A trusted endocrinologist who can be on call at all times should be part of your medical team.
- A "diabetes sensitive" obstetrician should also be part of your team (see Choosing a "Diabetes Sensitive" Obstetrician).
- A nutritionist should be available to you in case you need help adjusting your diet in the first months of pregnancy.

- You should be prepared to test your blood three to four times a day (depending on your doctor's recommendation) while you are trying to conceive.
- Like all women trying to conceive, you should be taking a maternal vitamin, which provides you with extra folic acid—important in preventing many birth defects.

CHOOSING A "DIABETES SENSITIVE" OBSTETRICIAN

Part of preparing ahead for pregnancy should include putting together a medical team to monitor your condition closely and to support you through your pregnancy. In addition to your gynecologist, your endocrinologist will be closely involved with your pregnancy. If you do not already have an OB-GYN, you may want to ask your endocrinologist for recommendations.

Generally, you'll want to pick an OB-GYN that specializes in high-risk pregnancies, which include not only the pregnancies of diabetic women but also those of any woman over 35. Rather than scaring you, having a doctor who specializes in high-risk pregnancies should assure you that you will get the best possible care during your pregnancy and that your doctor is aware of all the complications that may occur and able to cope with them successfully and immediately. Having such a specialist is the best way of ensuring that nothing does go wrong for you or your baby. You may also want to contact the branch of the American Diabetes Association in your area for recommendations of obstetricians and hospitals that will best accommodate your needs.

YOUR DIET

Calculating a diet that will meet your needs as an expectant mother and as a diabetic during pregnancy may be a little bit tricky at first. But, once again, your trusted Glucometer will help you through. Your doctor will probably also recommend that you work with a nutritionist at first, so he or she can help guide you toward finding the right number of calories and the right amounts of protein, fat, and carbohydrates.

During your pregnancy, it is even more critical than ever that you eat when you are supposed to eat. Consider mealtime to be as important as that last train out of the station that you just can't miss. Never skip a meal. Never skip a snack. Now, more than ever, it is also important not to cheat on what you eat. Remember that what you do or don't do has consequences for the health of both you and your baby.

When you are pregnant, you will need more calcium and more protein to meet the needs of the developing fetus. This fits well with your needs as a diabetic and will probably not disturb your blood sugar. Also, it will be important to eat small meals throughout the day and evening to avoid fluctuations in your blood glucose levels.

If you have maintained control of bgls with diet and exercise but are having trouble doing so during pregnancy, your doctor may want to suggest prophylactic insulin injections. In most cases, this would mean that you would use insulin for the duration of your pregnancy but be able to return to your old regime once you've had the baby. If your doctor recommends this course, by all means do it. You will be protecting your baby and yourself, and you may be able to avoid taking insulin in the future by using it prophylactically now, during pregnancy, when your pancreas is being taxed by the extraordinary process you are undergoing.

If you are insulin dependent, your needs for insulin will change during pregnancy, diminishing in the first trimester and then increasing until the third trimester. During your C-section, your need for insulin will be monitored continuously. Then after delivery, your need for insulin may drop once more. Throughout your pregnancy, you may also be at risk for insulin reactions. You should discuss your changing insulin needs with your doctor prior to conception and watch your blood glucose levels like a hawk. Think of planning your insulin needs as fine tuning a concert grand. It takes time and meticulous attention, but the result is well worth it.

Since the focus of this book is not insulin dependent diabetes, you may want to ask your doctor if there is any reading material he or she could recommend on diabetic pregnancies. You may also want to find a support group for pregnant women with diabetes to help you remain vigilant during pregnancy.

YOUR PREGNANCY ITSELF

If you maintain excellent control of your blood glucose levels, your pregnancy should be as normal as the next woman's. If you are an insulin dependent diabetic or if you are taking insulin for the duration of the pregnancy, you should know that the insulin you take does not cross the placenta. Glucose, however, does. For this reason, the babies of diabetic women whose control during pregnancy was not good, tend to be very large—almost always necessitating a C-section delivery. When control is tight, babies are normal size. Interestingly, in severe diabetics who may have vascular complications, babies tend to be very small. This occurs because such complications may restrict the blood supply to the baby via the placenta. Often, these babies need to be delivered early.

Other problems that may occur during a diabetic pregnancy include increased amniotic fluid (hydramnios). Hydramnios may make you feel very uncomfortable, and it may also cause your labor to be premature. The treatment for hydramnios is usually bed rest. If you have Type I diabetes and have been diabetic for a long time, you may also experience kidney problems and vascular problems. The possibility of such complications should be discussed thoroughly with your doctor before you decide to become pregnant. Toxemia is another possible complication that occurs less and less frequently during diabetic pregnancies as the number of women who maintain good control of blood glucose levels during pregnancy increases and the value of good control heads the list of recommendations by doctors treating diabetic women who are pregnant. Vaginal infections during pregnancy are common for all pregnant women. Your urine will be checked regularly for vaginal infections, but not for sugar. However, if you keep track of your blood glucose levels vigilantly with your Glucometer, you'll know of any fluctuations long before sugar spills over into your urine.

A HEALTHY BABY

When you've kept tight control during your pregnancy and if your pregnancy has reached term, your baby will be as healthy as the next baby, in all likelihood. Your baby will not be born diabetic and probably will not develop diabetes. In fact, there is only a 1 percent chance that your baby will develop diabetes if you have diabetes. (If both partners are diabetic, the risk is much higher.) If your blood glucose levels were somewhat high, your baby, in utero, will have responded by producing additional insulin. After the baby is born, your pediatrician will want to test your baby's blood to see if he or she needs a sugar supplement to neutralize the extra insulin. This is only a temporary condition. If your control was not perfect, your baby may also be at a higher risk for jaundice (high blood bilirubin), but in most cases, this is not a serious condition. Sometimes the babies of diabetic mothers are kept in the ICU (intensive care unit) for a day or two as a precautionary measure. This does not mean there is anything wrong. Your baby is just being observed, and you will be able to visit your baby in the ICU and even bring a blanket and a stuffed animal for his or her bassinet. If your baby is premature, he or she will require longer hospitalization in the ICU. In most cases, when control is good and your pregnancy has been closely monitored, you will leave the hospital with your healthy baby along with all the other new mothers.

UNDERSTANDING GESTATIONAL DIABETES

One day you go for your prenatal checkup and give your OB-GYN your routine urine sample, and suddenly she looks at you cross-eyed. Well, no, not really. But she looks at you with some, if not grave, concern. She tells you sugar is spilling into your urine—that little strip of litmus paper changing color is not a pretty sight. This is a symptom of gestational diabetes.

You will then be scheduled for a 1-hour glucose tolerance test, during which time you will drink a vile, sweet, thick, cola-like liquid that will pucker your lips with its too sweet taste, and you will wait while your blood glucose levels rise and a nurse tests your blood every hour on the hour. Depending on the results of this rather boring, time-consuming test, you will be advised to take insulin for the duration of your pregnancy, or if your bgl levels do not rise too high, you will be sent to a nutritionist to work out a meal plan to stabilize your blood glucose levels. It isn't really so bad. It happened to me.

I had a chance to manage my gestational diabetes through diet, and I followed my nutritionist's advice to the letter, eliminating even more borderline foods than she advised. Within a week, my blood had stabilized, but for the remainder of my pregnancy, I had to see my OB-GYN once a week. It was a good thing that I liked her and that we got along. My son, Dashiell, was born healthy and perfectly normal; he weighed 7 pounds at birth, smack dab in the middle of the normal birth weight range. If gestational diabetes is not controlled, birth weights may be abnormally high and a cesarean delivery may be necessary. I did have a C-section, but it was not related to my gestational diabetes. (I simply never dilated after 20 plus hours of labor.)

Gestational diabetes may also be referred to as maternal diabetes and is usually diagnosed at the beginning of the third trimester. A diagnosis of gestational diabetes does not mean that your baby will be born with diabetes. In addition, gestational diabetes is unlikely to cause birth defects, which usually occur in the first trimester. If you have gestational diabetes, you may give birth to a high birth weight baby, and a cesarean delivery may be indicated. In addition, your baby may suffer from hypoglycemia (low blood sugar) directly after birth. As long as gestational diabetes is treated quickly and appropriately, it need not cause any serious complications.

About 3 to 5 percent of pregnant women in the United States are diagnosed with gestational diabetes, and the American College of Obstetrics and Gynecology recommends the 1-hour glucose tolerance test for all pregnant women. Anyone may develop gestational diabetes, but there are certain risk factors, including being overweight prior to conception, a family history of diabetes, having given birth previously to a very large infant, a stillbirth, and being over 25 when you become pregnant.

Gestational diabetes occurs because the placenta produces a number of hormones during pregnancy to help preserve the pregnancy, and these hormones may block the production of insulin. The contra-insulin effect generally begins after the midway point of the pregnancy (between 20 and 24 weeks) because as the placenta grows larger, more hormones are produced, increasing the contra-insulin effect. When the pancreas cannot compensate by producing more insulin, gestational diabetes results and must be treated with a dietary regimen or with insulin injections. Once the hormones produced by the placenta are removed from the blood after birth, gestational diabetes generally disappears. It should be noted, however, that women who have had gestational diabetes are at higher risk for developing

Type II diabetes, and approximately half of women who have had gestational diabetes do develop Type II diabetes within 10 years. So, if you have had gestational diabetes, you should make practicing diabetes prevention a part of your life.

OTHER ISSUES FOR THE DIABETIC WOMAN

While diabetic women generally fair well in the sexual arena, their diabetes may affect their gynecological health and vice versa. The problems faced by a diabetic woman regarding menstruation, menopause, and gynecological infections are not insurmountable or even that complicated, as long as they are attended to. It is important to know the issues you might face so that you will be prepared to take appropriate action.

MENSTRUATION

While hormones other than insulin, such as estrogen, do affect blood glucose levels, the effect varies among women. I find little variation in my bgl readings when I'm expecting my period, but a friend of mine who is a Type I diabetic and uses insulin finds that her bgls sometimes plummet, necessitating an adjustment in the amount of insulin she is taking.

Once again, you are lucky to be diabetic in the time of the Glucometer. All you need do to arrive at your own cycle's unique relationship with your newly diagnosed condition is to keep track of bgls before, during, and after your menstrual cycle for a few months and share the information with your doctor as you go. If there is little fluctuation, your daily routine need not change when you are having your period. Depending on how much your blood glucose levels fluctuate, you may need to change your dietary routine when you are premenstrual and menstruating, or if you are on oral medication or taking insulin, you may need to adjust the dose during this time. If you manage diabetes with diet and exercise, but notice marked fluctuations during your period, you may want to discuss trying an oral medication, at least temporarily. In all cases, how you manage your diabetes during menstruation should be something you plan very closely with your doctor.

MENOPAUSE

If you are an insulin dependent diabetic, you should know that after menopause, your need for insulin will probably decrease. You'll be able to manage menopause well, as long as you have your trusty Glucometer a finger stick away at all times. As with so many other aspects of diabetes care and management, home blood glucose monitoring can change your life as you make your way through the "change." If not easy, menopause for you will be more easily managed than for a diabetic woman only 10 years ago.

For example, 10 years ago, a diabetic woman experiencing "hot flashes" would be unable to tell whether a bout of "the sweats" was due to her menopause or a hypoglycemic meltdown. Now, all she need due is stick in a test strip, prick, wait, and read her bgl. If her bgl is normal, well then, she has to stick out the hot flash or consider hormone therapy. If it's low, she can take measures to correct the situation.

If you are entering menopause and you have your diabetes under good control, it's a good idea to go back to your strict regimen for a while. This means checking your blood throughout the day to see whether the variations in your blood sugar are the same or are changing throughout this period of hormone adjustment.

Since we know that hormones such as estrogen may affect blood glucose levels, you should consider hormone replacement therapy (HRT) very carefully with your doctor before signing on. If you have a risk of heart disease in your family, HRT may be worth the risk of a minor fluctuation in blood glucose levels. Once again, checking your blood regularly can be your guide. If you decide to take hormones and the fluctuation in your blood glucose levels is great, you can always quit.

As with menstruation and diabetes, the interaction between hormone changes and blood glucose levels will vary. To reiterate, every diabetic and, therefore, every diabetic's treatment is and should be unique. This is as true during menopause as at any other time of life. What is normal for you may not be normal for the next woman. And what is normal for you should be what works—this means what allows you to keep good control of your blood glucose levels and manage menopause without debilitating mood swings or uncomfortable hot flashes and sleepless nights. Once again, this is a time of life in which you'll want to be in close contact with your endocrinologist or diabetologist as well as your gynecologist.

VAGINITIS

Often diabetic women have a higher incidence of yeast infections. This occurs because yeast grows more rapidly in glucose. If your blood glucose levels have been so high that there is sugar in the urine, you've probably experience an extremely high incidence of yeast infections. In fact, many women discover they have diabetes after complaining to their gynecologist of chronic vaginitis.

Eating yogurt with active acidophilus cultures has been shown to lower the incidence of yeast infections. Of course, you'll want to choose plain yogurt to avoid the sugar in the fruit or other flavoring. You might also want to consider taking acidophilus tablets, which will have the same effect without the calories.

Once you begin to manage your blood glucose levels, you will probably have fewer bouts of vaginitis. Keeping your urine "sugar free" is the best way to prevent yeast infections—just one more motivation to take charge and take control of your diabetes before another day goes by.

part 3

Prevention,
Permanent

revention may be a buzzword of the '90s, and it may taste like castor oil going down by now, but in the world of diabetes, it is tantamount to a cure. Following a regimen that protects against complications by normalizing blood sugar will not only ensure your health and increase your longevity but also protect you against the enormous medical costs that often accompany the complications of diabetes when it has been poorly controlled. Prevention is not only good for you, it's practical.

THE GOALS OF THE DIABETIC

- To maintain blood glucose levels within the normal range
- To work with your endocrinologist and support team to achieve normal blood glucose levels
- To respect the importance of diet and exercise in supporting the goal of normal blood glucose levels
- To compose an accurate diet for your individual needs that takes into account new findings stressing the importance of reconfiguring the diabetic's diet to include a higher ratio of protein to complex carbohydrate
- To use oral hypoglycemic agents or insulin to achieve normal blood glucose levels if this goal cannot be achieved through diet and exercise alone
- To maintain excellent self-care in order to prevent complications
- To manage complications as soon as they arise with the help of your doctor

- If insulin dependent, to work with your endocrinologist to find the right insulin doses for your individual dietary and lifestyle needs
- To seek help whenever you feel you can't do it alone or when blood glucose levels spike at any time—to never hide from a problem, overlook a symptom, or postpone a call to the doctor because you are afraid of the consequences—and to remember that denying the issue will only make matters worse
- When taking OHAs or insulin, to remember to hew to your diet and exercise regime and not "cheat" because you think you can "get away with it" and to remember that diet and exercise are always of paramount importance for the healthy diabetic
- To let others know about the extraordinary strides that are being made in controlling diabetes and help other diabetics maintain a positive attitude and achieve positive results
- To remember, always, that diabetes is as individual as each of us and to work with your endocrinologist to find the customized treatment plan that works for you
- To never forget that every diabetic can do a little bit better and that's what counts

9

Diabetes Doesn't Kill You— the Complications Do

Diabetes can kill you, of course. A friend of mine died of a diabetic coma in his early 60s—he was alone and had been unable to manage reasonable blood sugar control. Sometimes he would forget to take his insulin. Sometimes he skipped his appointments with his endocrinologist, and he never talked about adjusting how much insulin he was taking. He was also blasé about his diet. By the time he died, he was already suffering from complications, including neuropathy, arising from years of poor control. He was a wonderful man, a kind man, and was a brilliant writer. You might say that when it came to his diabetes, he'd given up. I loved him, and I miss him. I'm not asking to have been diagnosed sooner, but I keep thinking that what I know now might have helped him then.

Yes, people do die of diabetes, but only after years of poor control and the advent of the life-threatening complications that eventually result in death. You have the opportunity, however, through tight control and proper self-care to minimize this risk. With good control, diabetics can end up dying as gracefully from old age as the next octogenarian.

There is no such thing as a life free of complications for anyone. However, as a diabetic, you have the opportunity to achieve what is impossible in life in general—that is, creating a life free of complications, at least in one area. And, as you'll get tired of hearing, a diagnosis of diabetes by no means condemns you to the complications further on down the road.

Remarkably as it may seem, the connection between tight control—keeping that blood sugar in the normal range—and a lowered risk of diabetic complications was not universally accepted until quite recently. Imagine that doctors actually debated the possibility of a connection between chronically high blood glucose levels and complications. Imagine that recommending keeping blood sugar as normal as possible was in question. It seems impossible that a disease, the first consequence of which is chronic hyperglycemia, or elevated blood sugar, would leave any doubt about the goal of treatment—normalizing blood glucose levels and keeping them there. It makes you want to say, "it's the blood sugar stupid." But so goes the evolution of medical treatment, which, like everything in life, isn't perfect.

Fortunately, as we know, diabetes has gone from singing in the chorus of the opera of human diseases to being a diva proper. The complexity of the condition and the art of normalizing blood glucose levels and keeping fluctuations to a minimum have taken center stage. And the connection between keeping blood glucose levels normal and minimizing complications has been confirmed. And once again, home blood testing is instrumental in making this goal possible.

If you have been taking insulin for a while and have had chronic fluctuations in blood glucose levels, you can still prevent, or even reverse, certain complications. Doing so will involve restructuring your routine, with your doctor's help, to correct the amount and frequency of your insulin injections to work toward more consistent blood glucose readings in the normal range.

There are, however, serious complications that can accompany diabetes and that cannot be taken lightly. This is one reason you need to be under the constant care of an endocrinologist or diabetologist. Whether you see your doctor every month or less frequently will depend on your level of control. Any time you notice your blood glucose readings are running consistently high (or low, if you are taking insulin), you should call your doctor immediately, try to discover the reasons why and solve the problem. At every visit, your doctor will check your eyes, your circulation, and your urine to ascertain whether any complications are present. The complications that most frequently accompany long-term diabetes are neuropathy, eye problems (most commonly, retinopathy), heart attacks and strokes, kidney problems, and foot ulcers (a result of neuropathic damage). Seeing your doctor regularly and being vigilant about keeping blood sugar normal can help prevent these sometimes life-threatening complications.

NEUROPATHY

The simplest definition of neuropathy is nerve damage. While neuropathy can occur for many reasons, it is a common and often baffling complication in long-term diabetics or persons whose diabetes has gone undiagnosed for years.

Autonomic neuropathy—which usually occurs in association with diabetes—affects the autonomic nerves. The autonomic nervous system is the part of the nervous system that regulates involuntary vital functions—important ones, including the activity of the heart and glands. Autonomic neuropathy caused by diabetes involves, then, damage to the peripheral nerves. The greater the damage to the nerves, the more severe the complications.

Neuropathy is one of the most common complications associated with poorly controlled diabetes. It also alludes an absolutely accurate analysis, much like the disease itself. Symptoms may be mild, or they may be so severe that they cause pain in the extremities, abdominal pain, and sleeplessness. Other symptoms include numbness, itching, tingling—the sensation known as "pins and needles." Such symptoms may come and go; in severe cases, they may be almost constant.

The nerve damage incurred in neuropathic complications affects the nerves' ability to conduct necessary messages. It can also alter the nerves, which can result in chronic pain in the area of the damaged nerves. While the effects of neuropathy may be felt at any time, they occur most frequently at night. Some pain may be severe enough to require pain killers or tranquilizers. One of the curious factors relating to neuropathy is that it may come and go. You may find that a few months after your neuropathy is diagnosed, it improves on its own. Of course, the one way to make sure your neuropathy will improve and cause as little damage as possible is to control your blood glucose levels.

Neuropathy results when blood sugar has been elevated for a long period of time. The high amount of sugar in the blood damages the nerves so that they are unable to function normally. Neuropathy occurs most frequently in the feet and legs, but some people experience numbness in their hands and arms.

Sometimes neuropathy affects the eyes, causing double vision and pain. If you experience double vision, call your doctor. Usually, the situation can be corrected within 6 weeks. Neuropathy may also affect digestion, as the muscles of the digestive tract may not contract as rapidly as they once did. This results in digestive organs not emptying as efficiently. This condition is referred to as gastroparesis or delayed stomach emptying. In all cases, these complications can improve once blood glucose levels can be controlled consistently. Neuropathy may also result in problems having to do with maintaining an erection (see The Risk of Impotence).

Reversing Neuropathy

It seems remarkable that a consequence as severe as neuropathy can be reversed, but such are the wonders and mysteries of diabetes. Thus, with the right care you have the possibility of appearing, for all the world, as disease-free as someone without diabetes. It is a disease with a "sleight-of-hand" component. You are the magician, and the sleight-of-hand occurs when you learn all the tricks of your trade and use them to stay in tight control.

Unless your neuropathy went undiagnosed for years and is, therefore, severe, you can reverse the effects of neuropathy by maintaining normal blood sugars. If you have symptoms of neuropathy, the first improvement you'll probably notice is in the reduction of numbness in the hands and feet.

Depending on the severity and duration of your neuropathy, the return of feeling to your feet may occur quite rapidly, within as little as a month of normalizing your blood sugar levels

Other changes may happen more slowly, such as improvement in digestion (the reversal of gastroparesis— neuropathy that impairs the function of the stomach). Improved absorption in the digestional tract usually takes place over a period of years. Also, if you have been capable of only a partial erection and capable only some of the time and the situation is related to neuropathy, this, too, should improve over time.

Remember, however, that if you tend to waver in keeping good control, your neuropathic problems will return.

RETINOPATHY AND OTHER EYE PROBLEMS

Whenever I go to see my endocrinologist—which is now only twice a year instead of four times a year, because my control is good—I shy away from the eye exam. I always try to convince him to skip it. "Doc," I say, "you don't need to do this. You and I both know you don't need to do this because my control is so tight." He always says yes, he knows. But I'm the 5 percent group who have to endure the exam because 95 percent of the patients are not keeping such good control. I go along with him, because what else am I going to do? And because, of course, he's right. He's protecting me, and that's his job.

Having my eyes examined makes me squeamish. It does most people. And there's something about how precious sight is that makes considering the possibility of losing it quite haunting. Next to the horror stories of foot ulcers becoming gangrenous and limbs being lost, I think it is the loss of sight that frightens diabetics most. And, of course, it doesn't have to happen. Research has shown that with early diagnosis and good diabetic control, particularly in the first 5 years of the disease, your risk of eye changes and difficulties is minimal.

Additionally, if you have been diagnosed with Type II diabetes, your chance of developing serious eye problems as a result of diabetes is much less than if you have been a Type I diabetic most of your life. Finally, if your diabetes can be controlled with diet alone or with the help of oral agents, your chance of developing eye complications is less than that of a diabetic who is insulin dependent.

Yes, it is true that diabetes is still a leading cause of blindness in the United States. Still, your chances are better than 90 percent of never going blind. In addition, as the watchword of the evolution of diabetes treatment—*tight control*—becomes a reality for more and more diabetics, the odds of your going blind will be even less.

If, however, you have had diabetes for 20 years or more, certain vascular changes in the eyes may be almost inevitable. (We may assume that this fact is predicated upon statistics compiled on diabetics treated in the 1970s and 1980s—when tight control was not as well understood as a major component in successful treatment. Therefore, loose control of blood sugars was probably common among these patients.) About nine out of ten diabetics who've had diabetes for 20 years or more develop what is called background retinopathy. This condition involves changes in the retinas where light is received and then relayed to the brain for interpretation. Usually the condition stabilizes. Sometimes it even disappears, causing no vision problems at all. Among those who do develop background retinopathy, only about 5 percent eventually develop a more severe complication—proliferative retinopathy (retinitis proliferans). In most cases of proliferative retinopathy, blindness may still be prevented.

So, if you have been diagnosed with background retinopathy, don't give up, feel this is the beginning of your demise, or feel hopeless, and don't fall into the pit of fear howling, "I may go blind. I may go blind." Think of it as one more wake-up call you should heed. As with almost all aspects of diabetes, you have more control than you think you have— *as long as you take control.* And don't rationalize the news by saying, "Gee, I was taking such good care of myself. I must be the one exception to the rule that good control can prevent eye damage." Sure, some people who exert fine control may still develop eye problems, and some who live recklessly, with blood glucose levels going wild more often than not, may never develop eye problems. But, then, people get hit by lightning, too. *"When blood glucose levels are stabilized within the normal range, the risk of eye damage is minimal"*— that is about as close to an axiom as we need get here.

So, when diagnosed with background retinopathy, what do you do next? With the guidance of your doctor, follow the advice in the diet and exercise sections of this book as much as you can. If you have been taking insulin for a long time, you may still be taking what Dr. Richard Bernstein refers to as "industrial doses," which are wreaking havoc with your blood sugar and forcing you to consume truckloads of carbohydrates to compensate. If this is the case, you should work out a new regimen with your doctor, one that calls for smaller, more frequent doses and that will be more useful in stabilizing blood sugar.

If you still find yourself eating against your better interests or playing fast and lose with meals, and if, as a result, your blood sugar still seems like a runaway horse and you can't get hold of the reigns, talk to your doctor about working with a nutritionist who specializes in diabetes (see When You Need More Help). The point with diabetes is to never give up, because positive change is always possible.

HEART ATTACK AND STROKE

Diabetics account for a disproportionate number of Americans who die of heart attacks or strokes every year. By now you know what I'm going to say next. It doesn't take much to hypothesize that the diabetics in this category have probably not been exercising good and consistent control of blood glucose levels. When bgls are poorly controlled, a diabetic is far more likely to develop arteriosclerosis—and develop it earlier than the general public. In general, diabetics are twice as likely as the general public to have coronary heart disease and to have strokes—if the diabetes is poorly controlled. Tight control can change all this.

If you are diabetic and overweight, it is extremely important to lose weight. If you smoke, you must give up smoking. If you feel you can't, seek help. Nothing, except poor control, increases your risk of heart disease and stroke more than smoking.

When you maintain good control, you minimize your risk of heart disease and stroke. Following the diet and exercise regime recommended in this book will also help you lower your risk of heart disease and stroke.

COMPLICATIONS OF THE KIDNEYS

Complications of the kidneys usually occur only in cases of long-term diabetics with poor control. Complications occur because over time the capillaries that form the intricate network of the walls of the kidneys tend to thicken and become more porous. If not treated, kidney complications may lead to uremia and, finally, kidney failure, which can be treated only with dialysis. Other complications may occur because of high blood pressure or persistent urinary tract infections. Once again, if you notice any changes in urination—whether you are going more frequently or less frequently or experiencing itching or burning—you should call your doctor immediately. Early and vigorous treatment of urinary infections can help prevent complications.

Research has shown that diabetics who keep their blood sugar well controlled run little risk of long-term complications, and there is evidence that embarking on a regimen of good control when complications already exist may arrest further damage and even partially reverse kidney damage.

FOOT ULCERS

When neuropathy is severe, you may lack sensation on the bottoms of your feet. When you can't feel your feet, it's easy to injure them or develop sores from wear and tear without even noticing. Neuropathic ulcers may also develop under calluses and become infected. Any infection on the bottom of your foot can become serious if not attended to. Thus, paying particular attention to the care of your feet is an important part of your self-care routine.

A NOTE ON INFECTIONS

Infections are nobody's friend, but they can pose a greater threat to a diabetic than to others. Infections may take longer for you to recover from, and they may be more severe if your diabetes is not well controlled and, therefore, your resistance is less than it might be. If you are insulin dependent, the amount of insulin you need may also increase when you have an infection. Put bluntly, infections are a challenge for the diabetic and can threaten your tight control. They may even wreak havoc on your blood glucose levels, depending on the severity of the infection and on how well controlled your diabetes was before the infection.

The first thing to do when you get sick is to call your doctor. If you are controlling diabetes with diet and exercise alone, he or she may prescribe insulin injections for the duration of the illness, because controlling blood glucose levels is harder during an illness. Using insulin prophylactically during an illness may help prevent your becoming insulin dependent later on.

The most common complication during an illness is acidosis, which can occur whether or not you are an insulin dependent diabetic. Acidosis is a result of hyperglycemia, or too much sugar in the blood. Hyperglycemia occurs when not enough insulin is present to metabolize sugar. When this happens, the body begins to feed on itself for energy—burning fat and protein tissue. This process results in the production of acetone and other ketones, which are fatty acids that are then released into the blood. Ketones are also produced in excess during starvation. Essentially, when your body begins to burn fat as emergency fuel, it is starving. Eventually, acidosis results, which can lead to a coma. Scary as this sounds, the good news is that acidosis does not happen suddenly; it develops over a period of a few days. So if you call your doctor as soon as you notice the first sniffle coming on, he or she will monitor you for signs and symptoms of acidosis and intervene as soon as you recount any signs or symptoms. The first and most important sign that you are at risk is an abnormally high blood glucose reading. You may need to urinate frequently. You may then become dehydrated and extremely thirsty, and if you test your urine, you'll find that sugar has spilled into it. If you notice any of these symptoms, call your doctor immediately. If you don't, you will begin to feel abdominal pains and feel nauseated. These symptoms mean you are close to losing consciousness and need immediate medical attention. So, don't let things go that far. This is not the time to tough it out or take two aspirin and call your doctor in the morning. This is the quintessential time to get help.

A Check List for Sick Days:
- At the first sign of illness, call your doctor.
- Use your Glucometer to test blood glucose frequently—three times a day if your readings are normal; more if they tend to be high or spiking periodically.
- If readings are high and you are an insulin dependent diabetic, call your doctor. He or she may want you to increase your dosage of fast-acting (regular) insulin.
- If readings are high and you are non-insulin dependent diabetic, call your doctor. He or she may prescribe small amounts of insulin.
- If readings are high, test for acetone (ketones) in your urine. Call your doctor if they are present. He or she will probably prescribe fast-acting (regular) insulin injections every 2 hours until the blood glucose level normalizes.
- Drink fluids. Try herb teas, seltzer water, or diet sodas. Drink only a little bit at a time to avoid nausea.
- Always try to eat. When I had the flu, I lived on beef broth, which I was able to keep down. For some reason, the beef broth was more appetizing than chicken broth, but chicken broth is an equally good choice for a delicate stomach. Dry, whole grain toast is another possibility, or you might try dry wheat crackers or bites of plain yogurt.
- If you can't keep anything down, call your doctor.
- Check all medications for sugar content.

FEET FIRST

Diabetic or not, all of us take our feet for granted. Those precious appendages that literally take us everywhere are almost always ignored and almost never pampered. We might think nothing of indulging ourselves with a fine meal, but we almost never think of indulging our feet. Guess what? Now that diabetes has joined your litany of "self-identifiers," you have to indulge your feet.

For a number of reasons, caring for the feet is central to managing diabetes well. First, if you have had diabetes for years and not practiced tight control, the first evidence of this lack of control is often poor circulation in the legs and feet. Poor circulation, in turn, weakens the body's ability to fight infection, because the blood cannot carry an adequate supply of "infection-busting" white cells to the lower legs and feet. Thus, a problem as generally benign as athlete's foot, and any boils, cuts, or other infections and injuries, can become dangerous to your health faster than you can say *diabetes*. Poor circulation also

Caring for Your Skin

If you've maintained poor control of your blood sugar for some time, the effects may show on your skin. Diabetics with very poor control tend to have extremely dry skin that may be itchy in places and easily irritated. In fact, boils, inflammation around the nails, and other skin irritations are often a doctor's tip-off to test for diabetes. Unfortunately, such a diagnosis is not an early one, as skin changes occur only after blood sugar has been consistently high for a long period of time.

When diabetes is poorly managed, a host of skin problems may manifest themselves, including fungus infections, which may plague you between your toes or fingers, around your nails, under your arms, and in other moist places on your body. Vaginal yeast infections are more common in women, and yeast infections of the groin are more common in men. The sooner you gain good control of your blood sugar levels, the less likely you are to suffer such problems.

Long-term diabetics may develop "skin spots." These are little brown, bruise-like marks that appear on the shins. They don't hurt, but they are impossible to get rid off.

Insulin dependent diabetics used to suffer far more frequently from insulin atrophy around the area where injections

results in very dry skin, which can crack easily and, once again, open the way for dangerous infection. The highly coveted trick, of course, is to prevent all this from happening by attending to your feet as carefully and caringly as you would your face.

I don't mean to spin out too far a yarn about the Zen of foot care. Feet are not as pretty as tulips or lilies, or as fragrant as roses and gardenias. Feet are feet, and they serve us well. So it's worth it to serve them. Personally, I hate feet. You might say I have a reverse foot fetish. I don't think people should ever appear in public in sandals. I don't think people should take their shoes and socks off until it's dark and the lights are low. (You can imagine how I must avert my eyes on beaches.) And yet, since I started my foot care regime, even I have grown fonder of my feet. I still can't say I find beauty there, but I've come to respect my feet for giving me what I need, and I try to serve them well. And that is about as imperfectly Zen as the body gets.

Not only will caring for your feet protect you from diabetic complications, it also will be good for your feet, in general, and

are most commonly given. Because insulin is much purer today, this condition has become far less common.

The best protection you can give your skin is to get and keep control of your blood glucose levels. But there's no harm in taking extra care of your skin, even when your control is good. I have naturally dry skin, so I take heed and do the best I can. Here are some tips:

- Use a natural soap high in oil—aloe vera, avocado, or other high-oil natural soap. Avoid soaps with additives that may dry your skin.
- Don't use soap on your face. Use a natural facial cleanser instead.
- Rinse your face every night with cool water before applying your skin cream. This will aid in absorption.
- Take showers and don't scrimp on your shower soap. Use a high oil, natural soap on your whole body.
- Don't soak in the tub too frequently. This can dry your skin.
- If you do like baths, use a bath oil. But get yourself wet first. Then add the oil. Wet skin will absorb the oil more readily.
- Apply skin cream to damp skin to facilitate absorption.
- If you notice any sign of a skin infection, contact your doctor.

it can be a very pleasurable duty. Though your foot care regimen may seem like much ado about feet at first, you'll get used to it quickly. You will be investing in a good insurance policy that will protect you against unpleasant consequences for the long term, and your feet will thank you.

DAILY CARE

You should wash your feet every day. If you engage in rigorous athletic activity or wear sandals, or, heaven forbid, spend any time barefoot, you should wash your feet again. Washing your feet should become as accepted a part of your daily routine as brushing your teeth. Avoid deodorant soaps, which can be drying. Try to choose a nonalkaline soap instead. Nonalkaline soaps are least likely to dry your skin. Always test the bath water or shower with your wrist or elbow, not your foot (if you have lost any feeling in your lower legs or feet, you will be unable to tell if the water is hot, and you may burn your feet). Dry your feet well with a clean, soft towel. After drying your feet, use baby powder and a natural skin moisturizing lotion or cream. Make sure your moisturizer does not contain alcohol or any medication. To avoid the risk of athlete's foot, do not rub the lotion or cream between your toes.

YOUR PODIATRIST

As well as an endocrinologist or diabetologist, every diabetic should have a podiatrist. While you may not pay frequent visits to your podiatrist—if your control is good and you have no loss of circulation in your legs and feet—you still need to have a doctor whom you can call in an emergency. Usually your specialist will recommend a podiatrist to you, and even if your feet are perfect and perfectly lovely, you should pay the podiatrist a visit simply to establish contact and a rapport in case you need him or her in the future.

A podiatrist specializes in foot care and often knows more about the care of the feet and lower legs than your doctor. Your podiatrist is licensed to diagnose and treat disorders of the feet. He or she has completed a 4-year postgraduate program and received a degree of doctor of podiatric medicine (DPM). Make sure your podiatrist has this degree and comes highly recommended. If not, there are many podiatrists in the sea of feet.

PEDICURES

Pedicures have an on-again, off-again reputation in the world of diabetes and diabetes treatment. For most diabetics who are stable and not suffering from complications, pedicures are a great idea. First of all, it's a lot easier to have someone else trim your toenails, especially as you get older. In addition, the pedicurist is expertly trained in using small nail scissors and is far less likely to nick or scratch you than you would be. Add to that that he or she doesn't suffer from your own particular self-destructive tendencies to pick, pock, or gouge. All in all, the professional is the safer bet. And pedicurists do more than simply trim your toenails. They keep your calluses and corns under control, and . . . they massage your feet. This is good for your circulation, and it feels great too.

Make sure you are visiting a reputable pedicurist, and make sure you inform her or him that you are a diabetic. If you feel uncomfortable about any of the tools that are being used, ask to skip that part of the pedicure. Check to make sure the pedicurist is using tools that are sterilized.

I was already "into" pedicures before I was diagnosed with diabetes. I told my pedicurist about my diagnosis, and, low and behold, she told me that her mother is a diabetic. I've asked her not to use certain tools, and she completely understands. Now we trade notes on diabetes every time I'm there. She's great, and my feet feel great.

The Shoe Can Make or Break the Foot

As we neglect our feet, so, too, do we neglect what we put on our feet. From wearing shoes that pinch or cramp to wearing high heals or wearing shoes until they have no heals, few of us choose footwear as carefully and consciously as we choose the rest of what we wear. Now is the time for all of that to change.

Make sure you choose a shoe that fits every part of your foot well. Your foot is composed of twenty-six delicate bones and seventy-eight delicate and complex joints, all of which must be well accommodated by your footwear. The bones and joints of the foot take a lot of wear and tear, and damage to them can be cumulative as we age, if we do not pay close attention to the messages our feet send us via those first tiny aches and pains that we have a tendency to ignore.

Believe it or not, even the time of day can affect how your shoe fits. Your foot is largest in the afternoon, after taking you through the shank of the day, and this is the time you should buy new shoes. You should also stand up when your foot is being fitted, to make sure the shoe will accommodate all of your toes in their natural positions when your full weight is on your feet.

Once you have chosen your shoes wisely, take good care of them, replacing them if they become in any way uncomfortable or when the heels wear down. Wearing your shoes into the ground is not a good idea for anyone, particularly if you are diabetic. Nails in the sole may begin to protrude; tears in the shoe lining can cause irritation. In fact, it is a good idea to make it a daily habit to check the interior of each shoe before putting it on to make sure there is no injury waiting to happen in that dark interior. (I've done this ever since a mouse jumped out of my sneaker long ago as a Bohemian youth in Greenwich Village; that's one way to start a good habit.) Remember also to vary your footwear. Do not wear the same shoes every day. Your feet will suffer, and irritations may occur that could lead to infection, not good for diabetics.

SOCK SENSE

Your best sock choices are cotton or wool. Natural fibers, such as cotton and wool, allow your feet to breathe, and most people find them more comfortable than synthetic socks. Make sure your socks fit you, as well as your shoes. A sock that is to small or large can irritate the heel, toes, or ball of your foot, and irritation can lead to stronger stuff, like infection. Do not use elasticized socks. Also, check your socks for holes. At the first sign of a hole, toss your old socks and buy new ones. This is not an extravagance; it is a necessary part of your prevention strategy. Avoid stretch socks. Women should avoid pantyhose because of the elasticized waist, but if your diabetes is under tight control and your circulation is normal, you can probably wear pantyhose with a lightly elastic waist to work. Check with your doctor first. Don't wear them every day, and do take off your hose as soon as you get home. Garter belts are a no-no as well, although you probably don't have to tell anyone that after about 15 minutes on a Saturday night.

BAREFOOT IN THE KITCHEN OR ANY OTHER ROOM IS A NO-NO

The Spanish say, "Nunca diga nunca." The diabetic says, "Never go barefoot." And in this case, never means never. Going barefoot in the kitchen may not make you pregnant, but you might cut your foot and get a wicked infection—more than not good, for a diabetic.

From the moment you rise from bed in the morning to the time you yawn deeply and crawl into your bed at night, your constant companion should be a shoe or slipper of some kind. If all bedroom slippers make you laugh and think of boats or fuzzy stuffed bunny rabbits, buy a pair of charming, black slip-on Chinese slippers, anything to avoid the temptation of running barefoot through the bedroom to the bathroom. (Do not, however, wear a thonged sandal, particularly if you have any diabetic complications. The thong might irritate your skin.) Whether the shadow knows or not, from splinter to thumbtack, you never know what lurks on the floor. On the beach you should wear water shoes, sneakers, or rubber sandals. Many brands, such as Birkenstock, make amphibious sandals that can take you from sand to water practically and stylishly.

INCREASING CIRCULATION

You can help put your best feet forward by doing exercises to help stimulate circulation. Any and all exercise you do, from swimming to playing tennis to river dancing, will help improve your circulation in general. In addition, you should try to fit in a few easy, quick foot exercises on a daily basis, including pointing and flexing exercises, ankle rotations, and relieves— raising your heels off the ground and lowering them.

FOOT CHECK

I check my feet as carefully and religiously as I checked my son's head for head lice when it was epidemic at his school. You should check your feet and lower legs every day for any new cuts or scratches, athlete's foot, beginning corns, calluses, blisters, carbuncles, and bunions. All of these are incipient problems that should not be left unattended. If you can't see to save your life, then you probably won't be able to see to save your feet and should ask a family member to take a look for you—thanking them profusely, of course.

If you notice any irritation, redness, broken or peeling skin, bruises, or swelling, call your doctor or your podiatrist. Don't treat the problem yourself, and don't wait until tomorrow.

Following is a list of never-nevers:
- Never pick a hangnail, sore, scrape, or scab.
- Never cut your nails close to the quick.

- Never pick, dig, or scrape at any part of your toe, toe-nail, or cuticle with a nail file, scissors, pin, razor, or any other instrument.
- Never use any medications on your feet unless they have been prescribed by your doctor. (This includes everything from hydrogen peroxide and iodine to corn plasters.)
- Never give yourself a foot bath (or even dunk your feet in hot water), use a hot water bottle, or a heating pad.
- Never use a steam room, take a sauna, or have a whirlpool bath—too hot, hot, hot.
- Never let your feet get too cold.

While all of this might seem like too much to remember—or a lot of nit-picking over toes, metatarsals, and heels—as the song says, it will become second nature to you as time goes on. It will also serve you well as a wise investment in your future.

CARING FOR YOUR TEETH AND GUMS

Diabetics whose control is poor are more susceptible to periodontal or gum disease than the general public. Good control is one sure way of minimizing your risk of gum disease and further problems with your teeth and gums. Even if your control is excellent, you should pay particular attention to the care of your gums and teeth. As we age, we are all at greater risk for gum disease. And managing gum disease, whatever the cause, can be more complicated for the diabetic, as any infection can cause problems in terms of blood glucose levels.

Periodontal disease, also called periodontitis, is caused by bacteria in the mouth. Plaque on the tooth and around the tooth allows the bacteria to thrive. Thus, to prevent periodontitis and the first stage, gingivitis, you need to get rid of the plaque. This takes conscientious brushing and flossing and the use of an antimicrobial mouthwash. (Listerine is the best, and there are cheaper, generic varieties.) If your periodontal disease is advanced, your dentist can prescribe a mouthwash that contains the antibacterial ingredient chlorohexidine (two such brands are Peridex and Perioguard).

I've had gum disease for years, and it's not related to my diabetes, though my diabetes could make it worse if I don't act like a general regarding tooth and gum care. It's inherited and not related to my diabetes, though almost every diabetologist upon hearing about it would say "Ah, ha . . . " before he or she checked my blood sugar history. My father has had gum disease since I can remember, and he has extremely low blood sugar, though at the age of 82 he has other health problems that he would gladly exchange for diabetes. But, although my gum disease may be my own unlucky inheritance, it behooves me to take extra care of the situation to avoid infection and any worsening of the condition.

I see my dentist four times a year. She is aware that I am diabetic and takes precautions. That means that before I have even a deep cleaning, I take an antibiotic. You should too. Here are some other tips:

- Brushing correctly is important. Your brush should be dry when you apply your toothpaste. Begin to brush along the gumline at a 45-degree angle, brushing straight up and down or in a circular motion. Brush the "attic" and the "basement," that is, the interior upper and lower teeth. Be sure to do the same for the molars. Use a toothbrush that allows ready access to your back molars. Also, remember to brush your tongue. Brushing for anything less than 2 minutes is meaningless.
- Flossing is a means of getting to those places your toothbrush can't reach. Think of flossing as mountain climbing as opposed to walking on a straight road. Use the floss that is most comfortable for you—thin, thick,

waxed, unwaxed, flavored, or plain (unless your dentist suggests a specific floss). It's how you floss and flossing regularly that matter. Wind the ends of your strip of floss around your two index fingers and get down—that is, between your teeth. Make sure you wind the floss around the tooth in order to maximize your access to the plaque your toothbrush has missed. Flossing is an extension of brushing. If you don't do more than when you brushed, you haven't done anything. Massage, don't cut into your gums, and don't forget your molars, including the back ones.

- You should brush at least twice a day and floss at least once a day. Instead of less is more, more is better in this case. Flossing before bed is preferable. That way your teeth have a very clean night's sleep.

- Use an antimicrobial mouthwash twice a day. (Listerine is most often recommended.)

- See your dentist regularly (at least two times a year; more if you have gingivitis already).

- If you have to have any kind of dental surgery, make sure your diabetes is under good control beforehand, take antibiotics, and make arrangements for prophylactic insulin injections with your doctor, just in case.

- P.S. A new anti-gingivitis toothpaste has just been approved by the FDA and will soon be on the market. You'll know when. It will be advertised.

10

Medication, Alternative or Otherwise

INSULIN REACTIONS

While there is a very remote possibility that diabetics taking oral agents may experience an insulin reaction, insulin reactions are mainly a problem for diabetics who take exogenous insulin. If you are taking insulin, reactions may occur when your blood glucose levels fall below normal levels or if they drop suddenly from any level, for example, from 300 mg/dL to 100 mg/dL. It used to be that diabetics were told to eat sugar immediately when experiencing an insulin reaction, but, in fact, you can raise your blood sugar by eating something healthy, like an orange, rather than a piece of candy. What you need is the carbohydrate. Discuss the right solution to insulin reactions with your doctor.

Early warning signs include anxiety, headache, nausea, weakness, sweating, hunger, shakiness, tingling around the mouth, confusion, palpitations, and even inappropriate emotional responses. The epinephrine (adrenaline) released by your body to aid in raising your blood sugar level causes these physical responses and emotional changes quickly.

Reactions may be caused by a poor diet, skipping a meal, engaging in strenuous exercise without compensating by using less insulin and taking in more calories, or taking too much insulin by mistake. Periodic, mild insulin reactions do not do any permanent damage. If, however, you are experiencing insulin reactions frequently, something about your routine is off, and you should talk to your doctor about adjusting your treatment regimen.

You can almost always avoid insulin reactions by measuring your insulin very carefully, eating what you are supposed to eat when you are supposed to eat it, adjusting caloric intake (eating more complex carbohydrates) and taking less insulin when you exercise, watching for insulin reactions the day after you exercise strenuously, eating a snack before you go to bed to avoid nighttime reactions, and keeping close track of blood sugar levels with your Glucometer.

KETOACIDOSIS

There is one reaction that can happen to any diabetic, insulin dependent or not, and whether or not you are taking oral agents, and that is acidosis. Poor control, extreme stress, infection, or sudden injury can result in acidosis, which is a very serious complication if not diagnosed and treated. Eventually, acidosis can lead to diabetic coma. However, there is one blessing, acidosis doesn't happen suddenly, even in brittle diabetics. So there are always warning signs. As long as you take heed, you will be able to cope.

Too much sugar in the blood for too long causes acidosis, which is basically a reaction to prolonged high blood sugar or hyperglycemia. When there is not enough insulin available to metabolize the glucose in the blood for fuel, the body begins to burn reserve fuel, including its own fat. Burning emergency fuel has a side effect—the production of ketones or acetone. If this process goes unchecked, diabetic coma and eventually death may result. One of the early signs of acidosis is a fruity smell on the breath that resembles the scent of alcohol. If anyone thinks you've been drinking, just remind them you're a diabetic. (If you're an alcoholic, too, remind them you're a diabetic anyway and then get help.)

Fortunately, in this era of home blood testing, you can help reduce the risk of acidosis to a minimal level—that is, if you are consistent about checking your blood sugar. Even if your control is excellent, you should spot check your blood sugar periodically. I recommend choosing one day a week and testing your fasting blood sugar when you wake up. Then check 2 hours after lunch, 2 hours after dinner, and just before you go to bed. That's what I recommend. But actually, I check my blood sugar about every other day, whenever I feel a cold coming on, and whenever I feel particularly anxious, under stress, or lightheaded. It can't hurt, and seeing the normal numbers come up on the Glucometer is reassuring. The saying "Better to be safe than sorry" is particularly apt when it comes to diabetes. As long as your blood sugar is under control, you don't have to worry about acidosis. If it is not, you must be much more vigorous about testing your blood. Discuss your regimen with your doctor.

Of course, it is extremely important to know the warning signs of acidosis. If you are conscientious about using your Glucometer, you should never have the misfortune of having to experience them, but just in case, here they are:

- High blood glucose levels
- Dry tongue
- Dry skin
- A fruity smell on your breath
- Sugar in your urine (but with the help of home blood testing, you should never get this far)

If these symptoms are disregarded, abdominal pains, nausea, shortness of breath, and drowsiness and loss of consciousness will result. So heed any of these warning signs and, for that matter, any other physical changes you may notice, and get thee to your doctor. And if you are insulin dependent, take extra insulin. Remember that acidosis can be controlled.

ALTERNATIVE MEDICINE: SEPARATING THE WHEAT FROM THE CHAFF, SOMETIMES LITERALLY

Treating illness and disease with herbs and other homeopathic remedies is nothing new. In fact, the recent explosion

Of Ketones and Ketostix

There is ketoacidosis, and then there are ketones in your urine, and not all ketones in your urine are a sign that you are about to go into a diabetic coma. Ketoacidosis is a form of acidosis that is accompanied by the accumulation of ketones in the body. This occurs because of the faulty metabolism of carbohydrates and can be a complication for diabetics taking insulin (see Ketoacidosis; and Insulin Reactions). However, if you are a Type II diabetic and you take this new diet to heart and stick to it, your doctor may find ketones when he checks your urine at your next visit. This does not mean that yours is an incipient case of ketoacidosis and that you are on the verge of losing consciousness. The ketones in your urine are probably a result of the changes in your diet.

When my doctor found ketones in my urine, he said, "You're either starving yourself, or you are a Type I diabetic, and we have to watch out for ketoacidosis."

I said, "Thanks for the options, Doc." (It's so much fun going to the doctor. You end up with so many things you can worry about.) He sent me home to buy Ketostix and test my urine every day for ketones. After you've changed diapers for a few years, dip sticking your urine is nothing. In fact, every day I thought to myself, "This is how diabetics lived only a few decades ago"—and, by the time sugar spilled into the urine, they were already in trouble. I was grateful all over again for my Glucometer.

When you add protein to your diet and cut way down on carbohydrates, ketones may end up in your urine. This is because your body now has to look elsewhere for fuel (it had been coming from carbohydrates), which means it will begin to burn fat. A little burning of

of alternative remedies for everything from bunions and arthritis to heart disease and cancer is really a reiteration of ancient practices—a perfect example of the adage, "Everything old is new again." This said, it should be noted that in almost all cases there is no substantial proof that alternative medical therapies work in the treatment of disease. Or, more succinctly, while homeopathic remedies may relieve symptoms, they do not cure disease. An herbal remedy may relieve indigestion in a cancer patient undergoing chemotherapy, but it will not cure the cancer.

When it comes to diabetes, my philosophy is to use everything you can to get the results you want, but to do it with caution and in close consultation with your doctor. Work on your

fat is a good thing, but you don't want to do too much of it all at once. Or put another way, you're doctor isn't going to want you to. Unless she or he is quite sure you are a Type II diabetic coping with insulin resistance, your doctor will be worried about ketoacidosis. There is some debate about ketones in the urine. Clearly, changing your diet radically can create a mild case of ketosis that will not be harmful. However, diabetics need to be more cautious about this situation than others.

My doctor had told me to increase my carbohydrate intake—that my diet was too severe. When I do things, I tend to do them 100 percent (when I was younger, I had a pretty good track record as an anorexic). Give up carbohydrates, I said to myself, you bet. And here I was starving myself in a different way than an anorexic, but starving myself all the same. I added servings of legumes to my diet, more vegetables, a tad more fruit, and a half a piece of whole grain bread a day. I was afraid my blood glucose levels would rise. They rose about 5 points, but that was it. And within days, my Ketostix were coming up negative. I also started drinking even more water (I'd been sloughing off), which can help you avoid ketones in your urine. Low and behold, the ketones were gone. I did not gain weight. And I felt I'd entered a new stage of my treatment, one that allowed me to enjoy a few of those lovely carbohydrates that I had thought I would have to do without forever.

I do recommend keeping Ketostix on hand at home, along with your Glucometer, in your repertoire of first-line defense against any complications, pitfalls, or pratfalls in your self-care treatment.

diet, stay physically active, see your doctor regularly, if you need insulin, take it religiously, if oral agents help, take them. And investigate the options alternative medicine may offer, as long as you are aware these options don't constitute a cure and that some "alternative options" such as ginsing, can even harm you. Though ginseng is often touted as a cure-all for modern ills, it is one of the worst things a diabetic can take because it almost always raises blood glucose levels. If you are taking ginseng, stop. If you are contemplating it, forget it. If you doubt me, talk to your doctor.

One of the first caveats to consider when addressing alternative medicine is that there are no controlled, clinical trials that point to clear, positive results in terms of regulating blood sugar levels. In a phrase, it's all hearsay. The second caveat involves the American personality. As with all other offerings on the palette of self-improvement, many Americans look at alternative approaches to traditional medical evaluations and treatment as a quick fix, a sure and better thing. Nothing could be further from the truth. While techniques of alternative medicine might relieve symptoms or enhance treatment, they will never replace regular medical care and treatment, nor should they be seen as avenues toward an ultimate cure. Once again, we Americans tend to grab everything off the shelf and expect salvation, and this doesn't work.

Personally, I am very open to the possibilities of alternative medicine as an aid to my medical protocol but not as a substitute. As hard as it may be to cope with our insurance policies, getting an appointment with our doctors, and waiting and waiting for those appointments, modern medicine helps us, as long as we know how to use it well, ask the right questions, and demand the care we deserve.

My own experience with alternative approaches to treating diabetes has been that such remedies have made little if any difference and certainly do not provide an alternative to a well-managed nutritional plan and a consistent exercise regimen. I do drink blueberry tea, which may or may not help lower blood glucose levels. (Teas are much less risky than tinctures or pills, because they provide only a mild amount of the herb in question.) I also take CoQl0 enzyme (see Nutritional Supplements). Some studies show that CoQ10 may help in oxidative metabolism, which may help diabetics utilize oxygen at the cellular level. Then again, it may not. But taken in recommended doses, it has not been found to be harmful to your health. Since garlic has been found to be beneficial to your health across the board, I also make sure garlic is part of my daily diet. While I love garlic and love cooking with it, a daily dose of garlic means a lot of peeling and chopping and negotiating with my 7-year-old son regarding recipes. To ensure my clove intake is covered, I take a garlic supplement. My supplement of choice is Garlique, which is odorless. Check your local pharmacy or health food store for garlic supplements. I've also become a big fan of aloe vera juice, which I mix with seltzer daily to aid in digestion. Some people swear by the gel, but the gel is too much for me and reminds me of an ex-favorite slime-like toy of my son's called Gak. In my opinion, the juice is good enough. Aloe vera juice helps aid digestion and, therefore, the absorption of nutrients. It may also help control gastroparesis (delayed stomach-emptying), which is usually caused by neuropathy and which can affect blood glucose levels. Gastroparesis is more common in Type I diabetics. Whether or not aloe vera juice can significantly control gastroparesis and whether or not you suffer from this diabetic complication, aloe vera juice is good for your overall health, has no side effects, and is worth investigating.

My rule of thumb for all of the possibilities offered by alternative medicine is that if it's not harmful and has been found in reputable studies to have overall health benefits, then why not try it? I would, however, caution you to discuss all alternative medicines with your doctor, and to remember that as with any medications, you should never exceed the recommended dosages. Overdoses and side effects are possible and can be dangerous.

Take, for example, my own foray into zealous overtreatment with herbs. After all, I said to myself, they're herbs. What can go wrong? Plenty. I had a rather painful experience when I got involved with an odd combination of roots and herbs that was highly touted as a treatment for diabetes. I swallowed burdock root, slippery elm bark, turkey rhubarb root, and a host of other hopeful sounding roots and such, and boy did I get sick. And the potion cost me a great deal to boot. Nothing against these valuable roots, but once again, all these remedies are no substitute for your own custom-tailored diet and exercise plan.

Dr. Andrew Weil suggests that blueberry leaf tea *(Vaccinium myrtillus)* may have a mild regulating effect on blood glucose levels. The tea is safe to take. Try a cup in the morning and a cup in the evening for 3 months and see if you notice any improvement in blood glucose levels. I still drink the tea regularly because my blood glucose levels have been so steady. Although I am quite sure that my consistently normal readings are due to the accurately tailored diet that I follow, I am not taking any chances. If my bgl is even one or two numbers lower because of blueberry leaf tea, why not keep sipping? You can find blueberry leaf tea at your local health food store. While tinctures and extracts are available, stick with the tea, which is milder.

Herbs often used in the treatment of diabetes are bilberry, bitter melon, fenugreek, garlic, goat's rue, mulberry leaves, and olive leaves. While ginseng is also heralded by herbalists to treat diabetes, doctors recommend against it (see About Diabetes and Drugs). Not even herbalists, however, recommend herbs in the treatment of Type I diabetes.

The bottom line with herbs is that the manufacturers of these products are not required to conform to any standards. In fact, the labels on bottles may not even list all the ingredients contained in the preparation or remedy. Thus, dosages cannot be accurately tallied, and side effects may occur. Before you begin to experiment with any herbal medicines, you should talk to your doctor. If you feel any side effects, stop taking the medication. Before taking any herbal medicines, it is a good idea to become as informed as possible about herbs. Two excellent reference books about herbs are *Herbs of Choice* by Varro Tyler (Haworth Press) and *The Honest Herbal* (Haworth Press).

The way to approach the options regarding the treatment of diabetes via alternative medicine is with an open mind, but very carefully. Following are some other possibilities offered by alternative medicine that I have encountered and tried.

NUTRITIONAL SUPPLEMENTS

If diabetes has been poorly managed, vitamin deficiencies may result. Some of the most common deficiencies include vitamin B6, folic acid, vitamin B2 (riboflavin), magnesium, calcium, zinc, manganese, and certain amino acids. When you are diagnosed with diabetes, you should ask if you have any of these vitamin deficiencies and discuss taking a daily vitamin supplement and any further supplements your doctor thinks you should be taking. Once again, taking more than the recommended daily allowance (RDA) is not recommended.

B Vitamins

After the age of 50, levels of vitamin B6 in the body drop substantially, and it is after age 50 that Type II diabetes is most likely to occur. There is some evidence that B6 may reduce the need for insulin and help to maintain normal blood glucose levels. It is advisable to take a vitamin supplement that includes the recommended daily allowance of vitamin B6, whether or not such claims are true.

Coenzyme Q10

There is some evidence that CoQ10 may stimulate the production of insulin. Dr. Andrew Weil recommends taking 80 milligrams a day for 3 months to help stabilize blood glucose levels. Once again, because the evidence from the medical community and that from the alternative medicine community is positive when it comes to CoQ10, I take the recommended daily dosage (as long as I have the money to keep a supply in the house. It's not cheap.)

Vitamin C

Just like the beat Sonny and Cher so aptly sang about, when it comes to vitamin C, the debate goes on. Yes, no, more, less— around and around the experts go. When it comes to being diabetic, a deficiency in vitamin C may lead to degeneration of the insulin-producing beta cells of the Pancreas, but on the other hand, megadoses may be severely toxic in diabetics with renal insufficiency. Once again, taking the recommended daily dosage of vitamin C won't hurt you and may help you, as long as you take the bio ascorbate buffered vitamin C, which is absorbed more readily and is easier on your digestion.

Vitamin E

Vitamin E is considered one of the more important antioxidants and may be helpful in the prevention of vascular complications associated with diabetes. It may also have an anticlotting effect that may help to prevent premature atherosclerosis. Once again, if you take vitamin E, you should not take more than the recommended daily allowance (RDA).

Chromium

There is much debate about chromium and blood glucose regulation, and a debate is just what it is. No one has the answers. Chromium may help to stabilize blood sugar and improve serum lipid profiles. Claims have also been made that chromium may help the body burn fat, which has made chromium supplements a major fad among the chronic gym bag toting, ab building set at the gym and other quick fix shoppers at every health food store in every town.

If you want to try a chromium supplement, Dr. Andrew Weil recommends that you take 200 micrograms a day of the GTF, niacin-bound form. Once again, consult your doctor before incorporating any supplemental treatments into your daily routine. Since the amount of this trace element needed by the human body has yet to be established, toxicity and side effects are a possibility, so don't take any of the megadoses recommended on some brands of chromium supplements. Once again, avoid tinctures, since an accurate dosage cannot be titrated.

Magnesium and Potassium

Deficiencies of magnesium or potassium may cause a degree of glucose intolerance, though this has not been proven. And there is some evidence that potassium may improve insulin sensitivity. These are not "wonder minerals," and any use of supplements should be discussed with your doctor, as you know. The overlap here is that on this diet, you may initially not be getting enough potassium, since the major natural sources are orange juice and bananas—which are not on our list. Thus, you should discuss this possibility with your doctor and make sure your multivitamin contains enough potassium.

Zinc

Zinc is also said to encourage normal production of insulin, but it may sometimes cause complications.

Digestive Enzymes

Digestive enzymes, such as protease and amylase, may be helpful in the absorption of nutrients when the function of the pancreas is impaired.

In general, your vitamin and mineral needs as a diabetic will be served by a good nutritional supplement that your doctor recommends, and the jury is out on whether or not any further vitamin supplementation is effective in the treatment of diabetes.

Remember that no vitamin supplements or alternative treatments are viable substitutes for a healthy anti-diabetes diet and nutrition plan, accompanied by a consistent exercise program.

ALTERNATIVE THERAPIES

Chelation therapy

Chelation therapy involves using chelating agents administered intravenously to restore healthy circulation by removing the plaque from arterial walls. Dr. Garry F. Gordon, cofounder of the American College of Advancement in Medicine, has treated patients with diabetes with chelation therapy for 20 years and believes patients have fewer amputations, occurrences of blindness, renal dialysis, and other complications of the disease. Research is underway on chelation therapy for diabetics, but for now, it is considered a radical approach and should not be contemplated without being thoroughly researched and discussed with your doctor.

Oral chelators include garlic, vitamin C, zinc, and some amino acids such as cysteine and methionine.

Chiropractic Medicine

Chiropractic treatment will not in itself lower your blood sugar, but it can be beneficial to your overall health. The spinal column acts much like a switchboard for the nervous system, and the premise of chiropractic medicine is that by keeping the spinal column well adjusted, the interbalance of the central nervous system, autonomic nervous system, and peripheral nervous system is kept in equilibrium, and good health is obtained.

Every year, more than fifteen million Americans consult chiropractic physicians. There is little risk of injury, and various chiropractic adjustments can be beneficial in improving circulation and increasing your overall sense of "wellness."

Acupuncture

Acupuncture can alleviate pain and is said to increase immune response. Acupuncture uses special needles inserted under the skin into the "acupoints" (the thousand plus points within the meridian system said to stimulate the flow of the vital life force *qi*, or *chi*) to help correct and rebalance energy flow and, therefore, relieve pain and restore health.

Opinions on acupuncture vary wildly, although now the World Health Organization has listed 104 conditions for which acupuncture may be an effective treatment. While the cited conditions do not include diabetes, they do include addiction and obesity. If you feel you are "addicted" to sweets and/or if you are overweight, you may want to discuss the option of acupuncture with your doctor.

Reflexology

The basic tenet of reflexology is that there are reflex areas in both the hands and feet that correspond to every part of the body, including organs and glands. The theory is that by stimulating the appropriate reflex areas, stress and tension will be relieved in specific areas and, in the entire body, nerve impulses will normalize. Thus, overall balance will be restored. It's beautiful notion, but a tall order.

Some alternative therapists believe that reflexology with special attention to the points on the feet that pertain to the pancreas can help manage diabetes. There is no scientific proof of this. But reflexology certainly feels great. It can't hurt. It's great for your feet and can help improve circulation in your feet and lower legs, all important for the diabetic.

Massage and Circulation

Massage as a healing tool dates back to approximately 3,000 years ago, when it was used by the Chinese to treat a myriad of chronic conditions and illnesses. And Hippocrates, a Greek physician, espoused the medicinal effects of massage as early as the fourth century B.C.

Though massage is very popular in other areas of the world and is gaining in popularity here, many Americans still tend to be leery of getting a massage and of taking massage seriously as a way of improving overall health. The theory is that Americans are not the touchy-feely type, but it may also be true that many Americans just don't know what they're missing. This seems to be proven by the recent surge in popularity that massage has enjoyed in this country. Now, almost twenty-five million Americans have received at least one massage, and the number is rising.

If you are a diabetic or at risk for diabetes, massage is definitely for you. Think of it this way: The good news is

that you can no longer think of massage as a self-indulgence; you have to think of it as a necessity.

Firstly, massage definitely improves your circulation, which severe diabetes can put in jeopardy. Your skin is the largest organ of your body, and it contains about five million touch receptors. Amazingly, there are as many as three thousand receptors in a single fingertip. A full body massage works to trigger these receptors, which in turn can not only stimulate circulation but also lower blood pressure and even reduce the heart rate. Massage stimulates the brain's production of endorphins, which can improve your mood and also suppress pain, an added boon if you suffer from arthritis as well.

Secondly, massage stimulates the vagus nerve. The vagus is one of the nerves that influences bodily functions, and a branch of it connects to the gastrointestinal tract. And here it stimulates the release of the food-absorption hormones, including—you guessed it—

CHECKUPS AND FOLLOW-UP CARE

If you have been diagnosed with diabetes, your family doctor or internist probably diagnosed you. Once the initial diagnosis was made, he or she probably recommended an endocrinologist or diabetologist to you. An endocrinologist is a medical specialist who treats diseases and conditions of the endocrine system, diabetes being chief among these conditions.

Your specialist will play a very important role in helping you control your blood glucose levels and successfully managing

insulin. Thus, massage can improve food absorption, allowing you to receive the maximum nutritional benefit from the food you eat and, possibly, improving how your body processes glucose. And even if absorption improves only a little and not a lot, every way in which you can "de-tax" your pancreas is beneficial.

Thirdly, massage reduces stress. It does so by lowering the levels of the stress hormones called norepinephrine and cortisol. Less stress is good for diabetics and non-diabetics alike. In addition to simply improving your quality of life, lowering your stress level may help you stick to your goals and help you resist the temptation to indulge in old, now dangerous, comfort foods.

There are also some studies that show that massage helps to boost the immune system, which can help to lower your risk of infection. But whether or not this is so, there is enough evidence that supports the benefits of massage for everyone, including diabetics. And if that's not enough, don't forget that massage has no calories, is far less expensive than even a short vacation, and is a great pleasure.

In addition to a full body message, you might try reflexology and dry massage. Reflexology involves massage of the hands and feet. While there is no evidence that reflexology can refurbish your pancreas, it makes your hands and feet feel wonderful and is certainly good for their circulation.

Recently a friend gave me a pair of fairly odd looking knit gloves. The color was nice—a pale turquoise. The material was an odd, almost scratchy synthetic. I was not impressed. Then she explained the function to me. Dry yourself after your shower and rub your skin toe to top to improve circulation, stimulate energy, and keep your skin healthy. If nothing else, it wakes me up in the morning. And as long as you don't have severe complications, it can't hurt.

your diabetes. So you should choose your endocrinologist well; the better your relationship with him or her, the stronger your resolve and motivation will be in keeping blood glucose levels steady and living well with your diabetes. Next to your family and close friends, your specialist is the most important member of your diabetes management team.

Depending on the severity of your diabetes, you may see your specialist as often as once a month or as infrequently as twice a year. Try not to change, skip, or cancel any of your appointments. With so much time elapsing between appointments, we all have a tendency to forget the time and date, particularly when the appointment in question is one with a doctor that you may not be looking forward to seeing with great anticipation. Many specialists send reminder cards, since forgetting appointments is more common than not. But to ensure that you're there when your supposed to be there, write your appointment down in your daybook as soon as you make it.

In addition to seeing your specialist regularly, you should be vigilant about the rest of your medical care as well. When diagnosed with diabetes, you should inform your dentist, optometrist, and any other specialists you see regularly. Your overall health can be affected by your diabetes, and anyone who treats you should be alerted to this change in the big picture regarding your medical profile.

Because I've been getting good results and it's always nice to get praise wherever and whenever, I've actually come to enjoy my appointments. I'm also fond of my doctor, and we've developed a good rapport over the years. If you do not have a good rapport with your doctor, consider changing doctors. Perhaps he or she was helpful initially, but you feel you're not getting the care you want now. That's okay. Situations change, and you can change doctors. Remember, you're in this for life; you may as well make it as easy on yourself as possible.

LONG-TERM ADVICE

Always consult your endocrinologist or diabetologist if you become ill or have an infection. If you are planning surgery, consult your doctor. If you must have emergency surgery, inform every caregiver that you are diabetic and, of course, always wear your MedAlert bracelet. If you are planning on becoming pregnant, you should meet with your doctor, who will help you find a "diabetic sensitive" OB-GYN (see Chapter 8, Pregnancy and Diabetes). If you notice any dramatic changes in your blood glucose levels or if you notice a slow but steady rise in your levels, contact your doctor. For that matter, if you notice any metabolic changes, skin changes, any bleeding of the gums, or anything irregular in your overall health, you should be in touch with your doctor. Prudent attention now can help prevent complications later. .

part 4
The Art of the Diet

Americans are obsessed with food and, therefore, equally obsessed with dieting. It's like some unrecorded Greek paradox that some unsung, unknown, or unborn philosopher forgot to hand down—stuffing and starving will always go hand in glove. He or she who gobbles with the left hand will find the right hand always picking through the calories, fat grams, and nutrients for a theory of weightlessness that does not exist. And he or she who eats at the table is condemned to search forever for the unholiest of grails—a fad diet that will work. At this point, there are diets that are designed around your "color sense," your blood type, and your astrological sign. Where do we start? Where do we stop?

When it comes to food, the truth is that we need it, all of it—fats and protein, as well as complex carbohydrates. Our bodies depend on food for energy and also for vitamins and minerals. We also need water to keep the system flowing smoothly. In fact, poor old innocent water is about the only non-incendiary, non-politicized nutrient in the picture. All the experts agree we need it, and strangely enough, most of us still don't drink enough of it. But I'll save that saw for later. What the experts don't agree on is the answer to this question: "What is a balanced diet?"

Let me do a little debunking here. I recently finished an in-depth section on nutrition for a major medical guide. What I learned in researching everything from portion size to desired daily calories from protein was this: Nobody has the answer, which is to say, there is no answer. There is only balance. I won't go so far as to say nobody knows anything. But after reading reputable analyses by award-winning medical doctors, I would conclude with another philosophical tidbit: Two opposing ideas can coexist and cause consternation for an entire population. Low fat, high fat, high protein, no protein, all carbohydrate, ban carbohydrate—all roads lead to this: We need all nutrients. We need proteins, fats, and carbohydrates, probably in that order, though I don't want to say I know more than somebody else. And let me stress that getting a smaller percentage of daily calories from a nutrient such as fat does not in any way lessen the importance of fat in the diet. Look at it this way. The calories from fat are that much more potent and powerful, so you need less. And the calories from carbohydrate have recently been over-rated. Combining the percentages of our calories to comprise our daily caloric intake from this triumvirate has become tricky for us diabetics, but not impossible.

Recommended percentages in this plan will always be approximations—and as long as your percentages fall in a reasonable range of the recommended, if always vacillating, you're doing okay. Food is not mathematics. Try as you might to weigh your skinless, boneless chicken breast and get a perfect, 3-ounce piece, you will probably be at least a microgram off to the left or right of your appointed portion size, because food does not go lightly into equation form. In any case, such precise calculations are fit only for committed obsessive-compulsives and those who don't want to "get a life," as the cliché goes.

And the food lore and fad propaganda for diabetics is all the more confusing. One day it's say yes to carbohydrates. Then it's say no to carbohydrates, and yes to protein. But here is where you, the diabetic, have the edge. You have a barometer that absolutely won't fail you—your blood glucose reading. Using your blood testing kit to monitor how the combination of foods you eat affects your blood glucose levels will make balancing your soon-to-be-balanced diet easier. And if it works for your blood sugar, it works for you.

11

Getting Started on Your Food Program

When it comes to eating, as a diabetic, you have two equally important needs—to keep your blood glucose levels in the normal range and at the same time, to maintain a healthy, well-balanced diet that will meet all of your nutritional needs. This balancing act can get tricky. You may become so intent on keeping blood sugar low that you become obsessed with a restricted, even extreme, diet and so deprive yourself of essential nutrients. Such a diet may begin to cause other health problems that will, in turn, aggravate your diabetes. Or you may work hard to keep carbohydrates to a minimum to manage your diabetes, but in reality, you may be storing up your "carb" allotments to spend them all in the wrong place—sweets, confections, and other sugarplum fairy delights. You already know such indulgences do you no good, but stripping your calorie intake of all the good things—like vegetables, fruits, and legumes—will only make your health worse and increase your risk for heart disease, osteoporosis, and certain forms of cancer. Don't let this make you wail and weep. Not only is life not easy, it gets harder as you age, whether or not you have diabetes. Crying in your cotton candy won't help.

What will help is realizing that the only good diet is a balanced diet. This holds true for everyone, diabetic or not. What will also help is realizing that the nutritional plan you set in place now will serve you your entire life, protecting you from disease and boosting your immune system, as well as regulating your blood glucose levels. In fact, the healthy diabetic's diet is a diet that can improve even the non-diabetic's health. So, if all else fails, all you need do is remind yourself that even if you were not diabetic, a balanced diet is of the utmost importance to overall good health. This means that a diet high in a variety of proteins and complex carbohydrates, with a modicum of fat and a negligible amount of simple carbohydrates, including refined sugar, is the right diet for you and the caloric altar at which you ought to be worshipping anyway. You're not being deprived. You're enhancing your life.

Nutrients and Calories

Of the six nutrients, only protein, fat, and carbohydrate provide calories for energy, and the amount varies. Alcohol also provides calories, but these are considered "empty" calories, since alcohol is not a nutrient.

- Fat = 9 calories per gram
- Alcohol = 7 calories per gram
- Protein = 4 calories per gram
- Carbohydrate = 4 calories per gram

By this listing, you might make the wishful deduction that carbohydrate is as good for you as protein, but don't forget that for you, lowering blood sugar is at least equally as important as lowering the number of calories you consume.

Other interesting calorie facts include calories per ounce of common foods:

- Vegetables = 5–10 calories per ounce
- Fruits = 15–20 calories per ounce
- Lean meats = 25–50 calories per ounce
- Bread = 75 calories per ounce (ugh . . . there you go, another reason to ban bread, at least at first)
- Pure fat = 200 calories per ounce (oops . . . but that's why our portions in this department are smaller)

POINT OVERWHELM

So you've got your diabetes, you've got your poundage problem, and you've got all this gobbledygook going around in your head about good fat and bad fat, high carb and low carb, protein this and protein that. You've also got your cholesterol problem, your high blood pressure, your osteoporosis, your cancer gene, your mid-life crisis, your mid-life baby—take your pick. And what you really want to do is just give up. It was too much before you had diabetes, and it's way to much now.

Remember, we don't come into the world simply as diabetics. We're human first, and all the rest results, including common falls, from the grace of self-discipline and resolution. The first thing to do is to forgive yourself. Then try to keep it simple. If you try to change everything in your life all at once, you will doom yourself to failure.

When you start to think you just can't cope with yet another thing, think of it this way. Cope with this one thing, and slowly; eventually other aspects of your new routine will fall into place. If you manage a diet that protects your blood glucose levels from rising sky high, you will, in turn, be managing a diet that manages your cholesterol level, blood pressure level, and a host of other issues that can become diseases. You might want to think of your "problem" (I don't think of diabetes as a problem, but a lot of people do, and a lot of people tell us that diabetes is a problem) as an all-purpose problem, the solution to which is an all-purpose solution.

ENOUGH OF EXCHANGES

Nothing against the old exchange policy, but it is truly the bane of any diabetic's existence and, in my own humble opinion, at least partially responsible for the terrible failure rate among diabetics when it comes to sticking to "the diet."

The truth is that exchanges drive you crazy. They're like grams and percents, only worse. To live your life by the exchange policy, you have to become an acolyte worshipping the god of perfect substitution. Some of us are capable; most of us are not. But being unable to parse the exchanges sentence does not mean you're a failure. You can lead a perfectly healthy, normal life as a diabetic without ever once uttering the word exchange (unless you're trading a summer house with someone in France) or calculating how many exchanges make a day, if not a summer.

All of this is true because of home blood testing. Home blood testing has truly revolutionized the treatment of diabetes and the way diabetics live. The Glucometer and other blood testing kits allow every diabetic to find out for herself or himself exactly what her or his pancreas can bear and what it can't bear.

THE ESSENTIAL NUTRIENTS

WATER

Water is the forgotten nutrient. Water is also the most plentiful substance in the body, so there is no excuse for forgetting about it. Though most of us have been admonished by everyone from our doctors to our mothers to drink a lot of the stuff, few of us drink enough.

This may help you change your mind about water: Water helps regulate body temperature. Water is instrumental in the conduction of nerve impulses, maintaining the immune system, digestion, elimination, and other bodily functions. Water also helps to keep the brain adequately hydrated. Whatever you think of your brain, you do need it to be adequately hydrated. You should also know that it takes only a 1-percent fluid loss for your body to become dehydrated. And a person of average weight and height who is in good health will lose about 2 cups of water daily, simply by breathing. Another 2 cups are lost through perspiration, and 6 cups are lost via bowel movements and urination. Obviously athletes and those who are extremely active or do manual labor lose an even greater amount of water during the course of a day. So start drinking—water, that is.

CARBOHYDRATES

Carbohydrates include sugar, starch, cellulose, and gum, but all carbohydrates are not created equal. The most important distinction in the world of carbohydrates is that between simple and complex carbohydrates. The rule of thumb is that sugars are simple carbohydrates, and starches are complex carbohydrates. But, in fact, all carbohydrates, whether simple or complex, are made up of simple sugars. The difference in the carbohydrate is due to molecular structure. As you might have guessed, complex carbohydrates have a more complex molecular structure. A complex carbohydrate is called a polysaccharide, meaning it contains more than two simple sugar molecules hooked together. Complex carbohydrates may contain a thousand glucose molecules or more. Obviously, such complex molecules take longer for the body to metabolize than the simplest sugars, or monosacharides, which are single sugar molecules and include glucose, fructose, and galactose.

Killer Carbohydrates: Fact or Fiction

Carbohydrates aren't really killers, that was just to get your attention, but they sure can damage your blood. They tax your insulin. They come at your pancreas in high gear, ready to become glucose immediately and with a vengeance. You might want to think of carbohydrates as the Jekyll and Hyde of foods. One's good. One's bad. But they are related.

Carbohydrates are broken down into two categories, simple and complex carbohydrates. The simple carbohydrates are the killers. These include white breads, pastas, and rice, and all sweets, as well as potatoes and almost all junk foods you can think of. These should be banished from your pantry and your diet, if not your vocabulary.

Carbohydrate Content of Some Popular Nonstarchy Vegetables

½ cup cooked of the following vegetables contains 5 grams carbohydrate and 2 grams of protein:

Asparagus
Bean sprouts
Beets
Broccoli
Brussels Sprouts
Cabbage
Cauliflower
Chard
Collard greens
Dandelion greens
Eggplant
Green beans
Green pepper
Kale
Mushrooms
Okra
Onions
Rutabaga
Spinach
Summer squash
Tomatoes
Turnips
Zucchini

1 cup of the following vegetables, raw, contains the same 5 grams carbohydrate and 2 grams protein:

Cabbage
Celery
Chinese cabbage
Cucumber
Endive
Lettuce
Parsley
Radishes
Watercress
Spinach
Tomatoes

Starchy Vegetables to Avoid:

Baked beans
Corn niblets
Corn on the cob
Lima beans
Most mixed vegetables (w/corn and cooked carrots)
Parsnips
Peas
Potatoes
Pumpkin
Yams/sweet potatoes

Bread and Cracker Products with 20 Grams of Carbohydrate per Serving:

Bread Products

Bread-white, French, Italian, pumpernickle, whole wheat, rye- 1 slice
Bagel, small
English muffin, ½
Biscuit, 2 inches
Bread stuffing, 3/4 oz.
Cornbread stuffing, 1/2 cup
Corn or bran muffin, small
Popover, small

Crackers

Animal crackers, 10
Graham crackers, 2.5 inch sq.
Matzo, 6 inch sq.
Melba toast, 5 thin slices
Oyster crackers, 21
Ritz crackers, 7
Saltines, 3
Triscuits, 5
Wheat Thins, 12

Because complex carbohydrates are digested slowly and efficiently, they provide the body with energy over time, unlike the "rush" associated with the consumption of simple carbohydrates or sugars. Obviously, every good diabetic knows that simple sugars are our worst enemies. They wreak havoc on blood glucose levels and should be on our most unwanted list.

As a diabetic, your relationship with complex carbohydrates may be as complicated as the carbohydrate itself. Some medical experts say yes to a high-carbohydrate diet. Some experts say no and recommend a diet that restricts consumption of complex carbohydrates severely. The American Heart Association recommends that 55 percent of total daily calories come from complex carbohydrates. If you are trying to keep your blood glucose levels stable and within the normal range through diet and exercise, this is probably too high. On the other hand, a diet that restricts your total daily calories from complex carbohydrates to 30 percent or less is probably too extreme and may cause dietary deficiencies.

The best way to ascertain what portion of your daily calories comes from complex carbohydrates is to trust your blood glucose readings. If you manage in the normal range at 40 to 50 percent, then this is not too much of a good thing for you. If you find your readings are high, cut back on your intake of complex carbohydrates, concentrating on eating beans and other legumes, lentils, and low carbohydrate bran crackers and cutting back on pastas and grains and whole grain breads.

PROTEIN

Protein is vital to tissue growth and repair. At present, protein rivals complex carbohydrates in the great dietary debates. Some experts think of protein as a "a bad-guy" nutrient and complain that Americans get twice the amount of protein they need. Others consider protein to be the new "good guy" in terms of overall nutritional health. One thing we know is true:

After water, protein constitutes the major substance in the body. So we may deduce from this that it is fairly important.

When digested, protein breaks down into amino acids, which are vital to the body's overall health. Nine out of the twenty-two known amino acids are called essential amino acids. Essential amino acids cannot be manufactured by the body and must be obtained from food. Animal proteins, such as dairy products, eggs, fish, and meats, contain significant amounts of all nine essential amino acids and are, therefore, referred to as complete proteins.

Adequate amounts of complete protein must be part of your daily calorie intake to ensure your overall health. The U.S. Senate Select Committee on Nutrition and Human Needs recommends 12 percent of your total daily calories should come from protein. This is equivalent to approximately 40 to 70 grams of protein per day. The American Diabetes Association recommends 20 percent of your daily calories come from protein. But many experts in the forefront of diabetes research believe these recommendations are too low.

Protein is a marvelous friend to insulin, as it is digested slowly and does not challenge your insulin with concentrated amounts of glucose to process. For this reason, as a diabetic, I consider protein to be one of my great friends. Approximately 30 to 35 percent of my daily calories come from protein, though not all of the protein I eat is animal protein. Other foods that are high in protein include tofu, beans and other legumes, and lentils, and these foods are almost always part of my daily diet. In addition, eating a high percentage of protein need not mean you are consuming an equivalently high percentage of fat. If 35 percent of my calories come from protein, probably 25 percent or less come from fat—and I try to make sure I'm getting the right kind of fat, in other words, almost anything but saturated fat. Since I don't like fried foods, I get a lucky break here, but don't be jealous. I've had plenty of unlucky breaks in life, so I try to make the most of the little lucky ones I do get. When I do eat animal protein, I tend to make low-fat choices, such as low-fat cheeses, low-fat cottage cheese, egg white omelets, fish, and chicken without the skin. I do, however, indulge in whole milk or half and half in my coffee, since these are lower in carbohydrate value than skim milk—amazing the things you learn when you read labels. So you see, it's all a juggling act. Throw your protein up in the air, catch your fat, and pass your carbohydrate on from hand to hand.

It should be noted that your protein needs are also determined by how active a life you lead. If you lead a sedentary life, you need far less protein on a daily basis than if you lead a very active life. I lead a very active life—walking everywhere, picking up after a young son—and picking up that young son, and I exercise rigorously almost every day. So as you work on your own customized nutrition plan, remember the more active you are, the more protein you need.

Now if you are a vegetarian in addition to being a diabetic, you must be sure you eat enough protein from other sources, since you don't eat animal protein. Legumes, such as soybean, lentils, chick peas, black-eyed peas, and other beans, may be combined with grains, such as oats, wheat, barley, cornmeal, and others to give you a protein-rich meal. If you do indulge in dairy products, adding a small amount of cheese to any dish will ensure you are getting enough complete protein. If you are diagnosed as a diabetic and are vegetarian, I suggest that you discuss your dietary philosophy with your doctor and perhaps consider modifying your regimen, at least until you make progress in controlling your diabetes.

FAT

Long maligned, fat, illustrious fat, is making a comeback. It turns out that fat, except for saturated fat, is not the villain it's been made out to be, but rather it is essential to overall health—a nutrient as good as any other, as long as the appropriate quantities are consumed.

The trouble with fat isn't fat's fault. The problem is that Americans abuse fat. We saturate our diets with saturated fats, namely butter, margarine, mayonnaise, most cooking oils, salad dressings, red meat, fried foods, and junk foods. And saturated fat is also hidden in many other foods we choose to eat every day.

Fats are composed of fatty acids or lipids, some of which cannot be produced by the body and so are referred to as essential fatty acids. The three types of fat are saturated fat, polyunsaturated fat, and monounsaturated fat. Saturated fat can raise total blood cholesterol levels. Fat is higher in calories than other nutrients. At nine calories a gram, your fat intake should be regulated in order to stay within your daily calorie limit, as well as

About Protein

Not too long ago, 1959 to be exact, a prominent physician, Dr. W. C. Rose, calculated that 20 grams of (high-quality) protein was all an adult needed to maintain good health, provided the adult diet in general was adequate. Before that time, Americans virtually lived on meat and dairy products. Slowly but surely, as the decades passed, the glories of the complex carbohydrate began to be sung. In the '80s, Carb loading became a watch-phrase for athletes. Oat bran was named the "magic bullet" when it came to heart disease. Pretty soon, fat was ostracized, with protein coming in a close second as the undesirable of the day. Vegetarian and vegan were in. Middle-class Americans began to study the worthiness of macrobiotics.

But while fads do come and go, the truth of the matter is that humans need protein and always will. And, we can't store protein, so we need it daily.

Now we have come full circle, though perhaps we are a bit wiser for all our dietary obsessiveness. Drs. Michael and Mary Dan Eades state that an average person needs approximately 70 to 100 grams of protein a day—a far cry from 20 grams. They also state that from a purely medical point of view, we do not actually need carbohydrates in our diet. In other words, our metabolic

to avoid the unhealthy effects of saturated fats. Diets high in saturated fats have been linked to heart disease and may be linked to certain types of cancer.

A certain amount of fat is necessary for a healthy diet. Fats help transport fat soluble vitamins and help facilitate the absorption of those vitamins. The cells of the body also use fat to produce hormones necessary to the regulation of many bodily functions. Fat also helps to keep the skin and hair healthy and is a potent source of energy for the body. This said, all of the work that fat does to keep us healthy can and is done by monounsaturated and/or polyunsaturated fats. While a very small amount of saturated fat provides essential fatty acids that we need, it is almost impossible not to eat enough saturated fat to meet this requirement. In fact, saturated fat should comprise no more than 5 percent of your daily calories.

needs can be met without including any calories from carbohydrates in our daily fair—a far cry from the message of the carb-laden diets of the '80s and early '90s. Of course, while in the abstract, survival without carbohydrates may be possible, no one is advocating such an extreme approach. No one is saying throw carbohydrates out with the bath water of the old dietary regime. The American diet is simply involved in a rebalancing act—as is the treatment of diabetes.

So, who do you trust? I trust Drs. Michael and Mary Dan Eades, Dr. Richard K. Bernstein, and, most importantly, my blood.

Not too long ago, it used to be said that too much protein could cause accelerated aging and disease and rapid deterioration in diabetics. Now the opposite claims are being made by experts. I can only agree. Using protein as the mainstay of my diet has kept me a healthy, drug-free diabetic for years now. One note of caution, however, is that if you have had diabetes for years and suffer from advanced kidney damage, this diet is probably not right for you (since the waste products produced when protein is digested must be excreted by the kidneys) and you should be following a diet prescribed by your doctor.

Not All Fats Are Created Equal

A rose may be a rose, but a fat is not necessarily a fat.

Recently, our culture has become so obsessed with fat, the villain, that we overlook the complexity of fat. Let's face it; some of this obsession with abstinence comes from the underlying truth that we love fat, we adore fat, we crave fat, and we long for fat as much as we long for love, maybe even more. Why is the French fry such a popular food? Fat. Why is a hamburger still more popular than Mom's apple pie? Fat. It wouldn't surprise me at all to discover that the lust for fat has replaced the lust for sex itself, in our collective libido. And guess why? We Americans are basically starving for the right kinds of fat, which makes us crave fats all the more. Read on to find out how to make fat a healthy part of your life and how to tell one fat from another.

To avoid taking a long detour into the world of fat, I'll put it simply: Americans eat too much saturated fat. To cut down on the saturated fat in our diets, we need to avoid whole milk products, fatty meats, and fried foods. However, I should note that I use half and half in my morning coffee because I consume so little saturated fat in general, and a little saturated fat is not a bad thing. It's only a lot that kills us. So make your choices sensibly.

In addition, Americans eat way too much of the omega-6 fatty acids and way to little of the omega-3 fatty acids. While both omega-6 and omega-3 fatty acids are polyunsaturated fats, low and behold, there's even a good guy and a bad guy in the world of unsaturated fats. The 3s are the good guys, and the 6s are the bad guys—well, not bad per se, but consumed in disproportionately high quantities compared to omega-3s. For optimum health, we need to alter the ratio so that we consume more of the omega-3 fatty acids and less of the omega-6s (see Sources of Omega-3 Fatty Acids).

What does this have to do with diabetes? Plenty. If you are overweight, too much saturated fat in your diet is probably part of the problem, and obesity is at least part of the reason for your diabetes. You need to cut back on that old devil, saturated fat. And studies have shown that omega-3 fatty acids can help in the maintenance of normal blood glucose levels—the mother of all goals for the diabetic. When you chew the fat, all you have to do is chew the right fat.

Sources of Omega-3 Fatty Acids

Now that you know what the right fat is, where do you find it? It's a little like dating. You've had your bad relationship—that is, with saturated fat. You know what you don't want. You know what you do want. Now, where do you find it?

Since this is not a book on the mysteries and glories of fat, but rather on being a successful diabetic, I'm going to keep it simple and tell you as much as you need to know to aid in your self-care of diabetes. If you want to know the whole story on fat you may want to read *The Omega Plan* by Artemis P. Simopoulos, M.D., and Jo Robinson. This excellent book will give you all the information you need regarding the types and quantities of fat you need in your diet to build your immune system and prevent disease. And, by the way, Dr. Simopoulos is very clear regarding the connection between the proper consumption of omega-3 fatty acids and the healthy management of diabetes.

In general, you will find omega-3 fatty acids in olive oil and canola oils, fatty fish, lean meat, most nuts (though nuts contain smaller amounts of omega-3 fatty acids), organically grown eggs from chickens that have been fed a diet high in omega-3 fatty acids, and the star of the show—*flaxseed oil*. To increase the amount of omega-3 fatty acids in your diet, eat fatty fish at least three times a week, make sure the eggs you eat are rich in omega-3, snack on walnuts, and embrace flaxseed oil. Well, don't embrace it, just include it in your diet religiously.

Fatty fish include the following:
- Salmon (all types)
- Tuna (packed in oil)
- Herring
- Anchovies
- Lake trout

Nuts to concentrate on include the following:
- Brazil nuts
- English walnuts
- Black walnuts

An Ode to Flaxseed Oil

Flaxseed oil is perhaps the unsung hero of the new fat revolution. It is one of the healthiest additions we can make to our diets to protect our immune systems, prevent disease, and help control existing conditions. And even a little is better than none. If you add anything to the staples you keep in your "fridge" after reading this book, let it be flaxseed oil.

The easiest way to make sure you are consuming an adequate amount of omega-3 fatty acids is to take a tablespoon of flaxseed oil straight every morning. I do this every morning before I drink my two glasses of water and have my morning coffee, but I'll admit that it's not a taste for sissies. I find the simplicity of taking it like medicine worth the odd aftertaste. It's only a quarter to seven, and I've done one good thing for myself. And I don't have to think about which nut, which eggs, what fish for the rest of the day.

If the taste of flaxseed oil is too much for your gentle palate, never fear; all flaxseed products will provide you with large amounts of omega-3, including flaxseeds themselves and products baked with flaxseed oil.

You can find flaxseed oil in the refrigerated section of your health food store. If you can't take it straight, try using it in cooking, in salad dressings, and in baked goods (only whole grain, of course). Ask whether your health food store has goods baked with flaxseed oil or write to the company that produces the flaxseed oil you purchase for further information. One respectable firm is Spectrum Naturals, Inc., 133 Copeland Street, Petaluma, CA 94952.

VITAMINS

Though they contain no calories and, therefore, cannot supply the body with energy, vitamins are essential for growth and the maintenance of good health. Vitamins assist in cellular, metabolic reactions in the body and are, therefore, referred to as catalysts. Vitamins are organic chemicals. This means they contain carbon. Most vitamins are derived from plants. Since most vitamins cannot be produced by the body, they must be obtained from the food we eat.

The thirteen essential vitamins are divided into two categories—water-soluble and fat-soluble vitamins. Water-soluble vitamins include the B vitamins and vitamin C. The fat-soluble vitamins are A, D, E, and K. Fat-soluble vitamins can be stored by the body for a much longer time than water-soluble vitamins, which means you need less of them. In fact, taking large doses of fat-soluble vitamins may have a toxic effect. Once a saturation level is reached, water-soluble vitamins are eliminated in the urine. So while taking large amounts of water-soluble vitamins may not jeopardize your health, it is a waste of money.

Many can play the vitamin market much the same way they play the stock market—with a lot of hope for great results and little common sense. And many Americans lose as much on their vitamin investments as they do on most stocks. In almost all cases, a healthy diet, rich in fresh vegetables and fruits, will provide you with the vitamins you need. It should be noted that while vitamins are essential for good health, they are only necessary in very small amounts.

MINERALS

Minerals are inorganic substances. This means they contain no carbon. Minerals are also essential to bodily functions and overall health and cannot be produced by the body. Like vitamins, only very small amounts of minerals are necessary in the diet. With the recent identification of many new minerals and microminerals, mineral supplements have become as popular as vitamin supplements, and the health claims and healing roles that they may play have been touted as nearly miraculous. Once again, playing fast and loose with mineral supplements can put a dent in our pocketbooks, while effecting no miracle cures, and may even cause serious side effects. The one exception is calcium. Calcium supplements are recommended for women to help prevent osteoporosis.

FIBER

We began with water, and we'll end with fiber—the invisible but essential bookends of a healthy daily diet. Like the maestro of an orchestra, you may not know exactly what she is doing with that baton, but you do know the orchestra would not be playing in harmony without that baton. Or put another way, if nutrients were states of mind, water and fiber might be considered as the unconscious, that underpinning that permeates all of the other states. Though not considered a nutrient, fiber does a great deal to aid the efficient absorption of other nutrients, and getting enough fiber is essential to good health. Also, some studies have shown that enough fiber may help to regulate blood glucose levels.

All fiber comes from the cell walls of plants. There are two types of fiber, water-soluble and water-insoluble fibers. Both are important in aiding digestion. Celluloses are water-insoluble fibers and are found in wheat bran. Lignin and hemicelluloses are also water-insoluble fibers and are found in whole grains and vegetables. While water-insoluble fibers do not dissolve in water, they absorb water. Absorbing water causes them to swell, adding bulk as the food in your intestines is being digested. This makes passing along waste easier for the intestines. Pectins are water-soluble fibers and are found in legumes and certain vegetables, as well as in apples and citrus fruits. Gums and mucilages are also water-soluble fibers and are found in legumes and oats. Water-soluble fibers may help in lowering cholesterol by binding with bile acids, which the body uses to pull cholesterol out of the bloodstream.

Americans, in general, do not eat fiber-rich diets, and guess what? Gastrointestinal and digestive ailments afflict almost half the population. Also, colon cancer is a leading cause of death in the United States. In fact, in all countries where fiber consumption is low, the incidence of colon cancer is nearly eight times that of countries where fiber consumption is high. As if that weren't enough to make you realize fiber is your long lost friend, approximately 100 million Americans suffer from constipation, a condition that can be readily corrected with a high-fiber diet. The American Cancer Institute recommends that Americans should consume between 20 and 35 grams of fiber per day. Most Americans consume only 10 grams a day. And many experts recommend that adults should consume between 30 and 60 grams a day. So start chewing.

For diabetics, fiber can be a particularly loyal and beloved friend and ally. *All fiber helps to slow down the absorption of glucose into the bloodstream.* Pectins and gums also slow sugar absorption. I know by now that I don't have to tell you what this means, but I will anyway, because it's so exciting. Fiber, that poor, unrecognized lowly relation, may help you keep your blood glucose readings steady and normal. I should stress that this has not been proven in clinical trials but that most experts agree that these properties make fiber particularly helpful to diabetics. As you increase your fiber intake, remember to do so gradually and drink plenty of water to avoid bloating, flatulence, and diarrhea.

CLIMBING THE FOOD PYRAMID

The food pyramid has been rebuilt, and while not a far, far greater thing for all of us, it is a somewhat improved guide to healthy nutrition. Diabetics need to heed the pyramid and make it work for them. The priority, on the one hand, is normal blood sugar levels, but at the same time, we don't want to jeopardize the rest of our health by being too extreme in that goal. It's a tough one. Paradox is the middle name of the diabetic and to some degree a synonym for *balance*—as in *you have to accept that you are different to manage in order to be similar.*

Let's face it; you can't possibly fill the bottom of the pyramid. Don't try. You're the same as anybody else, but to remain so, you have to eat a little bit differently. Portions of grains, legumes, and other complex and wonderful carbohydrates will play a small part in your life. It might be better to call it the food hourglass for us (see Chapter 12, The Diet Diary).

12

The Diet Diary: Your Personal Plan

It's about eating to live, not living to eat. It's about treating your diet as an ally, not the infernal enemy. It's about finding a plan that works for you for life, not going on one more diet. It's about using the food you eat to normalize blood glucose levels and keeping them normal, thereby making you a diabetic in name only, and about eliminating hypertension and lowering cholesterol levels in the bargain. And it's about starting now and sticking to it for the sake of your health and to avoid all those complications and expensive medical costs that will, otherwise, be waiting for you down the road.

There is a link between diet and heart disease, and there may be a link between diet and cancer, but nowhere in the story of human health and disease prevention is diet more intimately linked to health than in the case of the diabetic. Too bad that for years, out of ignorance, many diabetologists and endocrinologists were going about dietary recommendations backward, overloading patients on carbohydrates and leaving them starved for protein and fat (the good kind, of course). But it's a whole new ball game now. Whether you're newly diagnosed or have been a diabetic for a while, this diet can and will change your life for the better. Finally, the guidelines for a diet that will help the diabetic manage his or her condition without wildly fluctuating blood glucose levels are being established by research so that each diabetic has a better chance at a long and healthy life than ever before.

Unusual Suspects

Milk

Here's an odd fact. Milk is higher in carbohydrate content than half and half or cream, and skim milk is higher in carbohydrate content than milk. So, if you're used to a glass of skim milk in the morning, trade it in for some cream in your coffee and a tall glass of water.

Diet Foods

Remember, you're not on a diet; you're on a health sustaining regimen (don't expect help from diet foods anyway). Diet foods are a quick fix American phenomenon, the spandex of food—the creation of illusion being the selling point. Foods labeled "sugar-free" are foods that do not contain table sugar. However, there are almost two dozen other forms of sugar that may be substituted for table sugar. These include carob, corn syrup, fructose, glucose, honey, lactose, molasses, sorghum, and treacle, among others. So, if you were counting on that carob-flavored candy bar instead of chocolate, I'm sorry to say, forget about it. In addition, diet foods, even if they are free of sugar, tend to be composed only of fast-acting carbohydrate—like that

"fat-free, sugar-free" coffee cake you were depending on. So stay away. (If you feel bereft, see Sweets for the Sweet Deprived.)

Artificial Sweeteners

Just because they don't contain table sugar, doesn't mean they don't contain any sugar. Check all labels. If you see the suffix "-ose" in the ingredients, run in the other direction, or at least walk away. Saccharin is okay. Equal tablets, which contain aspartame (not packets, which contain glucose), are also okay. Stevia is also okay. It's sold only in health food stores, and it contains no sugars of any kind. That's about it, as far as I know.

Rice and Pasta

Oh those mainstays of the high carbohydrate way of life, how they raise your blood sugar. Even if your health food "expert" tells you that they're complex carbs that are digested slowly over a long period of time, don't believe him or her. Giving up rice and pasta will put you on the fast track toward significantly lowering your blood glucose levels.

You'll need to come to terms with a diet that pleases your tastes and enhances your health so that you can stick to it over time, a long time, say forever. Start slowly. Get yourself adjusted. Then make incremental steps toward solidifying a healthy daily plan, say over 6 months to a year's time. Don't go for broke and begin to fluctuate just like the yo-yo or binger/purger that so many of us become when bitten by the dieter's bug. This is not a diet in the way advertisers use the term to lure you into buying product, system, or drug; this is a diet as from the Greek "a way of living."

To sketch the plan in broad strokes, you need to concentrate on eating more protein and monosaturated and polyunsaturated fats, fewer complex carbohydrates, and on eliminating simple carbohydrates from your diet.

BEFORE YOU START

You'll need help, not just from your medical and personal support team. Your quasi-bibles should be *Protein Power* by Michael R. Eades, M.D., and Mary Dan Eades, M.D., *Food Values of Portions Commonly Used* by Jane Pennington, and *Calories and Carbohydrates* by Barbara Kraus. Particularly if you are Type I diabetic, you should also purchase *Dr. Bernstein's Diabetes Solution* by Richard K. Bernstein, M.D.

YOUR DAILY STRATEGY

Each diabetic has his or her own idiosyncratic way of processing glucose, and each of us has to work within the parameters of our own system. Therefore, we each must shape a dietary plan that works for us, that keeps blood glucose levels normal or close to that, and that provides us with the nutrients we need. I have a theory, however, that for me works in practice, and I'd like to share with you.

It goes like this: Start small, and start your day with protein. Then add on the complex carbohydrates as you go—in snacks, at lunch, at dinner. I'd say get bigger as you go, too, but I don't want you to think that by the end of the day you should be eating a meal fit for a sumo wrestler. Think of your body in the morning as a machine that needs to warm up. There's not a lot of digesting going on. Things, in general, have slowed down. If you load on the carbohydrates now, in the person of a couple of slices of toast or a bowl of cereal, you're shocking your pancreas into action. You're asking for a surge of stage one insulin and, therefore, risking a higher blood glucose level, if you are insulin resistant or if you don't have enough beta cells pumping away. If you eat protein, you're taxing your system less—letting it start slow and get into the rhythm of things. This means breakfast consists of eggs, eggs and ham, cottage cheese, or cheese on a bran cracker or other low-carbohydrate cracker, but if it works, it works. Try it and see.

Then at snack time or lunchtime, add your vegetables (later on beans or other legumes, but don't go overboard on

A Short List for Starters

If all the things that you have to do to change your life and managing your diabetes seems too complicated and too overwhelming and makes you want to run in circles and scream and shout, try implementing the following eight great tips to get you started on improving your life:

- Eliminate all refined sugar products.
- White out white—eliminate white bread, white rice, white pasta, and potatoes. These simple carbohydrates can be as perturbing to blood glucose levels as refined sugars.
- Eliminate fruit juices and choose fresh fruit instead.
- Eliminate junk food, and if you can't, at first, read the labels on snack foods to find the lowest in total carbohydrate content. Substitute whole grain products in moderation.
- Never overcook your vegetables. The fiber or roughage breaks down in an overcooked veggie, and in addition to being of little nutritional value, this tasteless, crunchless morsel you are eating may raise your blood glucose level because it is metabolized as glucose more quickly. You might as

the portion sizes). At dinner, if you have a glass of wine (to stimulate digestion), you will also stimulate insulin production—if only a little bit. This is a perfect meal in which to incorporate low-carbohydrate fruits, such as cantaloupe or strawberries, as a dessert. By now your system is revved up and your relatively normal blood glucose levels should be the proof of this "protein for starters" pudding.

YOUR INDIVIDUAL PLAN

Your daily target should consist of a 40-percent protein/30-percent carb/30-percent fat ratio. Remember that these are ballpark percentages. Nature didn't mean for mathematics to be the center of our diet. Nature designed food and the whole process of eating so that we can get the right nutrients.

Here's how to hit your target:
- Make protein the mainstay of your diet. Forty percent of your daily calories should come from protein. This

well be snacking on a simple carbohydrate, but don't.
- Stay away from soups and stews. The same principal holds true for soups and stews that holds true for overcooked veggies. As the nutritional value and the roughage component dissipate, what's left is a gluey substance ready to go straight to glucose, and fast. So do your insulin a favor and skip soups and stews. There are better meals to be had.
- Have two, small, high-protein snacks between meals to control your hunger and bgl levels.

- Eat less; eat more often.
- If you are overweight, create a weight loss program with your doctor that you can stick to.
- If you are sedentary, move. Any exercise is better than none. Take the stairs. Park further away from the office or shopping center and walk. Walk instead of taking the bus. Take the dog for a walk. Work in the garden. Pace while you are talking on your portable phone. In a word, move.

means __ grams to __ grams, depending on your size and body type.

- Minimize your carbohydrate intake, particularly during the first week of the plan. No more than 30 percent of your calories should come from carbohydrates, and this means complex carbohydrates. Depending on your size, this is equivalent to between 30 to 40 grams.
- Concentrate on eating the "good" fats (see Not All Fats Are Created Equal). Don't go over your allotted percentages, but you need not become obsessed with gram values as long as you stick with healthy fats.
- Keep it simple. If grams and percentages drive you batty, count on portion sizes to steady you and keep you in your target range. Protein per serving equals 3 to 4 ounces; carb per serving equals 1 cup steamed vegetable or salad greens. Check your bran or whole grain cracker package for portion size. Fat per serving equals a tablespoon of olive oil or other oil high in omega-3

What Should Never Pass Your Lips

I know it's hard. Each piece of the puzzle of managing diabetes is harder for some of us than for others, because we all have different habits, vices, and needs. But the sooner you simply restrict certain foods that blow blood glucose levels sky high, the sooner you will be able to get on with your own good life.

For all the research that has changed how we look at diabetes, define diabetes, and treat diabetes, one thing that has not changed is the pure sugar curse. The best way to cope is to just give it up.

The following is a list of non-nutritional items, still called food, that you should shun as you would the boyfriend or girlfriend who didn't call you back after ten embarrassing calls on your part.

- All candies, even supposedly sugar-free candies (They still contain sugar. It's just not table sugar.)
- Gum, except for some sugarless gum (Check the label to make sure the gum is not sweetened with glucose or any other "-ose." These are off limits.)
- Artificial sweeteners, except for Equal tablets, saccharin, and Stevia

fatty acids, an ounce of cheese, and so on. Remember, as long as you concentrate on eating the right kinds of fat, you don't have to worry too much about your percentages. You'll be eradicating so much saturated fat from your diet that you'll be in good shape vis-a-vis fat.

- Drink lots of water—8 glasses or more a day.
- Remember to count carbs and calories from snacks in your total.
- Start an exercise plan that includes a major anaerobic component.
- Eat before you are starving. Never let yourself get too hungry. That's when the cheating starts.
- Eliminate artificial sugars, except for Equal tablets and saccharin, and Stevia (if you can find it in your health food store).
- Eliminate all desserts, except sugar-free Jell-O.
- Avoid starchy vegetables.

- Cereals (When your blood sugar has been well controlled for a while, you may be able to have a small unsweetened bowl of a multigrain cereal, but, in general, stay away.)
- Chocolate (Sorry!)
- Desserts (except for sugar-free Jell-O)
- Diet foods (These foods don't contain table sugar, but they do contain other sugars and sugar substitutes that will raise your blood sugar.)
- Dried fruits
- Honey
- Fructose
- Fruit juices
- Instant breakfasts
- Protein drinks (Most of these contain a lot of sugar.)
- Jams, jellies, and preservers
- Maple-sugar flavored sausage or bacon
- Molasses
- Raisins
- Sodas, except for diet sodas (Make sure the diet soda you choose does not contain fruit juice.)
- Sugar
- Sweet wines
- Syrups
- Yogurt, except for plain yogurt (The brand lowest in carbohydrate is Erivan.)

- Eliminate all high-carb snack foods, such as chips of all types and popcorn.
- Eliminate all fruits, at first (eventually you can add small amounts of strawberries and cantaloupe).
- Include one glass of wine daily (3 grams of carbohydrate), if you wish, but don't forget to count the carbs.
- Check your blood glucose level four times daily—upon rising (before breakfast), 2 hours after lunch and dinner, and at bedtime. If you exercise, also check your blood before and after your work out.
- Don't get depressed if your bgls don't come down right away. If you stick to it, they will come down.
- If your blood glucose levels begin to normalize after 1 month, begin to add more complex carbohydrates, such

Cravings and Consequences

Everyone craves something that's not good for them some of the time, and everyone indulges such cravings more or less of the time. The trouble the newly elected diabetic encounters is that indulging a craving for something sweet or for the ultimate in starchy junk food may have a greater consequence than just a thousand extra calories, a sense of discomfort, and an evening of guilt. Your nasty delectable can wreak havoc with your blood sugar, havoc you don't need.

Try to avoid what you know to be your most tempting temptations. If it's fast food that brings you to your knees, avoid fast-food restaurants. If the smell of croissant drives you wild, don't go to the bakery. Never think of dining out as an excuse to indulge in foods that are not on your plan. The carbohydrates

don't magically disappear because a waiter has served you. Also, if you crave a starchy snack and do indulge, keep in mind your blood sugar will rise rapidly and substantially—say 30mg/dL or more, depending on the snack and depending on the individual.

The following tips may help you get a grip on cravings:

- *If you indulge anyway, test your blood within the hour*. Perhaps the evidence will help you resist temptation next time.
- *A half a whole wheat donut is better than a whole one*. Train yourself to appreciate a smaller portion size and refrain from going back for more.
- *Eat slowly*. Gobbling carbohydrates taxes your pancreas immediately

as legumes, lentils, and whole grain bread, to your diet—slowly and in small amounts, say one portion per day. Check your blood regularly to see if there is any deleterious effect on glucose levels.

It's important to take the following precautions:
- Don't undertake your new dietary plan without the supervision of your doctor. Consult your doctor whenever problems arise.
- Take a multivitamin recommended by your doctor.
- If you smoke, quit.
- If your blood glucose levels do not come down, talk to your doctor about oral hypoglycemic agents, insulin, or both.

and all at once. If you nibble slowly, you may do less harm, and you may eat less, too.
- *Don't count on fat-free snacks.* Check the calorie and carbohydrate value first.
- *Keep healthy snacks on hand.* Having something healthy on hand to nibble on can help you curb the urge to indulge.
- *Eat when you're hungry.* If you let yourself get too hungry, you're much more vulnerable to cravings.
- *Reorient your taste buds.* Make a concerted effort to try new tastes—perhaps a different cheese, exotic spices, dips for vegetables, flavored coffees to help steer your taste buds away from what they used to crave and toward delicious, new taste

sensations that won't raise blood sugar.
- *Add some unsaturated fat to your diet.* Many people crave saturated fat because they are not eating enough of the right kinds of fat. Make sure to include olive oil and/or canola oil in your diet, avocados, low-carb nuts, fatty fish, and other foods that contain monounsaturated and polyunsaturated fats. This can help curb your appetite and satisfy some of your cravings.
- *Cheat a little, not a lot.* In this case, even if less isn't good, it's better than more. Two tortilla chips will not do to your blood sugar what thirty will. If you say, "Poppycock. It isn't cheating unless you cheat a lot," then try not to cheat at all.

PHYSICAL CHANGES

You might find yourself getting thirsty on this diet, so keep drinking plenty of water. Initially, you may also feel slightly less energetic than usual, because you've cut the carbohydrate content of your diet. This will pass quickly. In the meantime, an extra half a cup of coffee can help.

You may also experience some changes in your bowel movements. Adding protein to your diet may constipate you temporarily (good reason for taking Metamucil). On the other hand, if you are eating more roughage than you are used to, this may lead to a bout or two with diarrhea or soft stools. In either case, your body will adjust quickly. If changes in bowel movements persist, you should consult your doctor.

YOUR PERSONALITY AND THE PROGRAM

As I've said, ad nauseam by now, just about anyone with a modicum of will can do better with diabetes. The hurdles in your way are your own resistance, the inevitable deflation or even depression that goes along with realizing you've got to cope

Yes, We Have No Tomatoes

Having declared an unreserved homage to vegetables, let me now say that not all vegetables are innocent. In particular, watch out for carrots. A cooked carrot does no one good and does a diabetic harm. Raw carrots are not much less suspect, but can be picked at in a salad without too much harm. Tomatoes are also a surprise enemy, sweet and starchy as they are.

The following is a list of the guilty parties:

- Beans, except green beans (for the first few weeks)*
- Beets
- Carrots
- Corn
- Peas
- Potatoes
- Tomatoes and tomato products
- Yellow squash
- Yams and sweet potatoes

with a lifelong condition and feeling overwhelmed by the challenge you envision to be before you.

To help you avoid sabotaging yourself, it's important to deal honestly with yourself about who you are when it comes to facing a challenge. Do you start fast and then fall apart before reaching the stretch? Do you do best with moderation in all things, including change? Or do you sit at the edge of the pool for hours, wondering whether or not it's worth it to jump in? You can make headway in regulating your blood glucose, whatever category applies to you, even if on bad days you count yourself a member of all three groups.

1. *The fast starter:* If you don't rely on food for comfort, don't have a major sweet tooth, and are highly disciplined, you'll probably manage the first 2 weeks of the extreme regimen I adopted fairly well.
2. *The medium starter:* If the program leaves you feeling bereft and overwhelmed by what you have to give up, if you think it isn't a day without bread and butter, you'll do better on a moderate attack plan in which

*A Note on Beans: I love beans—black beans, kidney beans, cannellini beans, aduki beans, fava beans. They're good for you. They can be used in many different dishes. And you'll see that they're included in more than one of my recipe tips. But when I started on the path to normalizing blood sugar, I did not eat them, because of their high carbohydrate content. So, I'm recommending that tip to you, with the proviso that once you've normalized blood sugar consistently (say for a couple of weeks), you try adding a small serving of bean salad to a daily meal and see what it does to your blood sugar. If your blood sugar stays relatively the same or rises only a few points for a short while, add beans to your list of acceptable foods. Beans, like nuts, are a complex carbohydrate that is digested very slowly, which means they may have less effect on your blood sugar than the same value carb that is digested more rapidly. So don't give up on beans; just put them aside for a while. They're an excellent source of roughage, and a good source of potassium, aid in digestion, contain an adequate amount of protein, and if you like 'em, they taste good.

your carbohydrate intake is 5 to 10 percent more. Try to restrict your carbohydrates to whole grain breads, legumes and lentils, and low-sugar fruits, such as strawberries and cantaloupe. If you manage your cravings with whole grain breads, you should be able to manage without pasta and rice. Your blood sugar levels will come down more slowly, but they will come down.

3. *The slow starter:* If you have the will, but just can't find the way, you'll need help. If you can't control your diet or just don't feel motivated enough to try, you may benefit from the support of a group such as Weight Watchers. Though their diet plan is not tailored to the diabetic's needs, you can modify your carbohydrate intake on the plan while gaining the benefit of group support. You may also need to take oral hypoglycemic agents to help lower your blood sugar. You may need to take them indefinitely, or if the progress you see yourself making inspires you to try harder, you may find you can manage good control without them within 6 months to a year.

The Cracker Barrel

Learning to love the "good" crackers is your best insurance against indulging in the breads that can drive blood sugar crazy. My "big four" are Wasa Crispbreads, Ryvita, Whole Grain Crispbread, Bran-a-Crisp, Wheat Bran Fiber Bread, and Bran Crispbread (the hardest to swallow, until you get used to the chewiness, but the lowest in carbs, since it's made from bran husks, not even the bran itself—and oh, what fiber). What follows is carbs per serving:

Wasa Crispbreads:
  8 grams—3 percent
Ryvita: 10 grams—3 percent
Bran-a-Crisp: 6 grams—2 percent
Bran Crispbread:
  5 grams—2 percent

The cardinal rule is keep carbohydrate value low, which all of these brands do. If you can't find any of these brands in your local market, look for whole grain crackers that are on sale and check the labels for carbohydrate value.

MY DIET DIARY

AT 1 MONTH

I was depressed. I felt I had lost a loved one. No, more than one loved one. Cantaloupe, strawberries, raspberries, no more, never? My lord, how hard can life be? Very hard. And not only those luscious, little fruits, but pasta too—the glue with which I stuck together any main course for a dinner party cum children? I was crushed. I was heartbroken. You mean I might see but never taste these loves again? This may seem like peanuts to you. Not peanuts, but eclairs, if you live for anything from Mallomars and Oreos and popcorn and bread and butter to lasagna and ice cream sundaes. Giving up these love affairs will be hard for you, no doubt. Perhaps impossible. If that is so, then you should try oral agents, but not until you've given giving up these bad habits a shot.

Diagnosis tends to make anyone desperate, initially. Then I began to think of all the other lovely tastes I wouldn't have to give up and might even be able to indulge in more—such as steak, butter, extra avocado, cheese, cream, and moderate amounts of wine. Sorrow notwithstanding, I was going to try.

My daily percentages of protein and carb are different now than when I was first diagnosed. During the first month, I almost eradicated carbohydrates from my diet completely. This was extreme, but I was determined to give managing my diabetes without drugs my best shot. I limited my carbohydrate intake to vegetables (those that were low in carbohydrate content) and green salads. I tried not to eat too much saturated fat, but I did allow myself steak for dinner whenever I felt like it and half and half in my coffee.

Legumes to Love

BRAND/TYPE	CALORIES	FAT(G)	FIBER(G)
Black Bean Soup (Bean Cuisine)	180 (1 cup)	5	7
Black beans (Progresso)	110 (1/2 cup)	1	7
Cannellini (Progresso)	100 (1/2 cup)	.5	5
Instant Black Beans (Fantastic Foods)	160 (1/3 cup)	1.5	7
Pinto Bean Dip (spicy) (Guiltless Gourmet)	35 (2tbsp)	0	4
Vegetarian Bean Chili (Health Valley)	80 (1/2 cup)	0	7
Vegetarian Beans (Heinz)	140 (1/2 cup)	.5	5

My menu went something like this:

- I started my day with a high-protein breakfast that included next to no calories from carbs. Usually, I had an egg white omelet. Sometimes, I had a half cup of cottage cheese with salt or a plain yogurt. If you add an artificial sweetener, use Equal or saccharin, which are made without glucose. Always check the label on an artificial sweetener and stay away from any artificial sweeteners that use glucose as the sweetener.
- My mid-morning snack was usually a ham "roll up"—a piece of ham with low-fat mayo and mustard.
- For lunch, I had fish—tuna fish if I was at home, something elegant and high in omega-3 fatty acids, such as salmon, if I was fortunate enough to have a lunch date. At lunch I tasted my first carbs, usually in the form of a salad with oil and vinegar dressing or blue cheese

dressing—sometimes low fat, sometimes not. I was not that concerned with my fat intake, knowing that a third of my calories could come from fat. I also had green leafy vegetables such as spinach or broccoli.

- In the afternoon, I snacked on a zucchini roll-up or a hard-boiled egg with low-fat mayo. Eventually, as my blood glucose levels started to come down, I added a handful of nuts.
- Dinner was a salad, vegetable, and protein dish, such as fish or chicken, and a glass of wine. I found a glass of wine lowered my blood glucose level just a tad, and so I would concentrate on having the major portion of my carbohydrate calories at dinner. This meant sometimes I treated myself to coleslaw (no carrots) or whole grain crackers (such as the Wasa brand) with soy butter or an avocado spread. I don't have much of a sweet tooth, so I didn't miss dessert. However, if you feel bereft without a sweet finish to your meal, you could have a bowl of sugar-free Jell-O.
- At bedtime (after checking my bgl), I had a slice of low-fat cheese, chicken, or ham, just to give my stomach something to do for the night.
- The first month I had almost no fruit, not even a taste. As my blood glucose levels came down, I added cantaloupe or strawberries (just a few at first) to my evening menu.

During the first 2 weeks, I tested my blood sugar often—usually four to six times a day, depending on whether I worked out or not. I tested my fasting blood sugar upon waking, before and after exercising, 2 hours after lunch, 2 hours after dinner, and right before bed. Literally within days, I noticed a marked and consistent drop—from 130–140mg/dL to 110–120mg/dL (the high end of normal).

Now, remember that I took an extreme stance and stuck to it. That might not work for you, and that's okay. You'll still make progress if you follow a modified plan that ups your protein intake and lowers your intake of carbs. What is most important is that you pick a level of the regimen that you can stick to. Remember, also, that I was motivated by that sword of Damocles. My doctor had said that if diet didn't do it, and quickly, I'd be taking insulin. I sing the praises of insulin. I knew how to inject myself. I would do it if that was what I needed to control my blood glucose levels, but I am one of those people who is "needle shy." There was no way of getting around my queasiness over the notion of a needle as a constant companion. Therefore, I used my irrational fear to motivate myself.

What I Did for Exercise

At first I stuck to my aerobic workout—about 40 minutes on the Stairmaster four times a week, plus walking 3 to 4 miles a day. Then I added an anaerobic routine, using a tape from a local New York City gym called "Crunch." I did my aerobic routine in the morning and found that my blood sugar was consistently high.

I decided to stick to walking long distances and doing my anaerobic routine in an all-out effort to manage my diabetes with diet and exercise. The rise in blood sugar caused by aerobic exercise was not all that significant. Still, I wasn't taking any chances. I know I should have increased the duration of the exercise, even if this meant I only had the time to work out two to three times a week. But hindsight is hearsay. I'm back to doing an aerobic workout three times a week: My blood sugar is under pretty good control, and because I work out for a longer period of time, the workout causes little or no increase in blood sugar (see Those Non-Identical Twins, Aerobic and Anaerobic Exercise).

What I Cut Out Completely

I ate no pasta, rice, bread, cereal, or grains (except for whole grain crackers) for the first 2 weeks of my diet. I eschewed all stews and soups, except for bouillon. I also avoided fruits, particularly those high in sugar/carbs, such as pears, grapes, and apples, and I skipped all fruit juices. The vegetables I relied on were all very low in carbohydrates. I didn't touch carrots, beats, tomatoes, or other high-carb veggies. My idea was to simplify, simplify.

Portion Sizes

My egg white omelets consisted of three whites and a yoke. Protein portions were approximately 3 to 4 ounces of meat, fish, or poultry. Snacks were approximately an ounce of low-fat cheese, 1/2 to 1 cup of cottage cheese, a cup of yogurt, or a slice of ham or turkey (about 1/2 an ounce). However, if I was hungry, I ate more. I wasn't worried about having a little more protein, since I knew that was not what would tax my insulin. I ate about a cup of broccoli, zucchini, green beans, or Brussels sprouts at any one sitting and a hearty portion of green salad. Once again, I wasn't too worried about portion size, since my carb intake was extremely low in any case.

WHAT HELPED ME THROUGH

I drank seltzer with a shot of natural lemon juice for a treat, and I drank plenty of water. I also had a cup of blueberry leaf tea every mid-morning. In the afternoon, I relied on my lemon-seltzer treat and chamomile tea. And, of course, I had my glass of wine at night (sometimes two), which accounted for a good-size portion of my carbohydrate intake—but was worth it in helping me feel I was not depriving myself. (If you loathe and abhor wine, you could add a piece of whole grain bread and butter, a portion of a low-sugar fruit, such as strawberries or cantaloupe, or a low carbohydrate dessert, such as a fat-free, chocolate yogurt—choose the brand with the lowest percentage of calories from carbs—usually 7 percent.) I took a complete multivitamin every day. Solgar is a good brand, but any reputable brand will do. I also took extra vitamin C, in buffered form to compensate for the lack of fresh fruits in my diet. By the way, I also drank copious amounts of water.

HOW DID I FEEL?

I was hungry at times (so I ate), a little headachy (so I took a Tylenol), and thirsty (so I drank plenty of water). Sometimes I had a peculiar taste in my mouth, due to the ketones produced as my body burned fat and the resultant mild acidosis. Diabetics used to high blood glucose levels often feel fatigued or just

The Final Word on Portion Size

We all know we shouldn't eat too much. Calories are as important to watch as grams of fat—and grams of carbohydrates for a diabetic. But how much is too much, and how can we tell what too much is? Well, there's no easy answer. If you are at all close to being a normal human being, human nature being what it is, you can probably safely assume that you should be eating larger portions of fresh vegetables and smaller portions of just about everything else, including steak, pasta, and desserts.

Fortunately, the new food labeling law has made our job a lot easier, which also means there are no more excuses.

Playing the Card Game of Portion Size (and Remember, You Can't Stack the Deck)

In general, you can assume that 3 ounces of fish, chicken, or meat is about the size of a regular playing card (as long as the piece that you're eating isn't 2 inches thick). You can assume that an ounce of cheese is equal to one half the card (once again, as long as your piece is not thicker than it is long). And a serving of pasta should be a little larger than a deck of cards, but not too much larger. Don't forget that if you pile your plate high or cheat in other ways, you'll be thrown out of the portion casino.

A Note on Restaurant Portion Sizes

In most cases, when you enter a restaurant, you are entering a funhouse when it comes to portion sizes.

strange when their blood sugar finds the normal range. Since my diabetes was diagnosed before my levels were through the roof, I didn't have such a reaction. I took Valerian root at night to aid my sleep. Placebo effect or not, it seemed to work. I did have some trouble sleeping, though. My doctor recommended Benadryl—the over-the-counter allergy medication—as a non-addictive sleep aid, and on difficult nights, I took two capsules. Since I no longer take it, my doctor must have been right. It is nonaddictive. (Benadryl does not affect blood sugar.)

If anything, I felt simple elation that my diet was working. In 2 weeks, my levels were down from the 140s to the 90s, usu-ally, with some readings between 100 and 115. Though I did not need to lose weight, I lost about 4 pounds, which, being an American girl, had the usual positive effect. Thin is still in.

Americans seem to remain convinced that there is an innate connection between quantity and quality, when, indeed, there isn't. And quantity can be dangerous not only because of the calories you are consuming but also because the more you eat at one time, the more taxing the job for your insulin stores and the greater the chances of higher blood glucose readings for more than a couple of hours.

Here's a list of just a few items to be wary of in restaurants:

	USDA Serving	Restaurant Serving
Bagel	2 ounces	4 ounces
Pasta	1 cup	3 cups
Meat	3 ounces	6 to 16 ounces
Salad dressing	2 tablespoons	4 tablespoons

And the list goes on. You can pretty much assume that you will be over served any carbohydrate, such as breads of all kinds, mashed potatoes, or French fries, which you should not be eating anyway. The best way to avoid temptation is to ask whether you can substitute a vegetable or a salad for your starch course. And a cardinal rule for dining out is that you never finish any course on your plate, except your vegetable dish.

One other thought: Often when I go out to dinner, I order two appetizers instead of a main course. The portions are smaller. There's greater variety, and I've just always thought the appetizers on most menus are more creative than the main courses. You can save calo-ries, keep your portion sizes in order, and enjoy a wide range of flavors and tastes this way.

My Daily Percentages

My percentages from protein, fat, and carbohydrate were approximately as follows (please note that all percentages are approximations—anything more exact is impossible for the normal, harried person to follow):

40 percent protein
30 percent fat
30 percent carbohydrate

To keep my fiber content up (and aid digestion during this radical dietary shift), I took Metamucil daily. It's natural. It's fiber. It helps.

Water, Water, Everywhere, and None of Us Drinks Enough

Mahatma Gandhi may have fasted for an extraordinary length of time, but he could not have done it without water. Water is the body's prime ingredient and most essential necessity. Though water has no food value, the body cannot survive for even a relatively short period of time without it. Water is as essential as any other essential nutrient to the body's well being, and it is the elixir of good health. Yet few of us heed the repeated admonishments from health care professionals and health publications to get our eight glasses a day of cool, clear H2O. Why even highly respected, world-class doctors that I have worked with have uttered such blasphemies as "Oh, why put that in the book, nobody can drink eight glasses of water a day." Well I can, and if I can, you can.

Start by drinking an eight ounce glass of water in the morning, before you have your coffee or tea. Without being too holy or new "agey," I find this can be one of those ordinary, quiet spiritual moments that people are now going through a lot of far-flung efforts and contortions to find. The first thing I do in my day is something that is absolutely, without reservation, good for me (unless there's lead in the pipes—but I'm hoping there isn't, and in a faithless world, you still have to have faith.) Without putting too fine a point on it, there is something purifying about a glass of plain, cool water. Of course, because I'm more a Type A personality than anything else, I add a few ounces of aloe vera juice so that I can feel I'm getting just a little more out of the experience. It's the American way. Then I lunge for my cup of coffee, feeling wholesome.

AT 2 MONTHS

Having triumphed—at least in terms of blood sugar, if not the rest of life—I began to play a bit fast and loose with my health. I don't mean that I indulged in a dozen glazed donuts or anything of the sort. No, no. I mean that I had the magic lamp—protein. Rub it, or more accurately, eat it, and you got your wish—lower blood glucose levels. Knowing this, I developed what might be called a form of dietary tunnel vision—fool's gold.

As long as kept my blood sugar within the normal ranges, nothing else mattered. I ate my protein. I had mesclun salads, because it was easy—grab a bag and fill it with the tongs at the local market or health food store, dowse it with a low-carb

How and when you manage your next seven glasses will depend on the work you do and your daily routine. Whatever you do, keep water nearby. If you work at a desk, keep a pitcher of water and an attractive glass on your desk, and keep the glass filled. Sip your water throughout the morning. Make sure you know the number of ounces the pitcher holds. Then when it's empty, you'll know how much water you've had. Then, fill it up again. If you go to the soda machine, buy a seltzer instead. If you go out to meals, remember to request water, and drink your glass of water before you drink any other beverage or start eating your meal.

It should also be noted that water is particularly important when you are overhauling your diet, as you are doing now. When you add roughage to your diet, increase the amount of protein you are eating, and decrease the amount of carbohydrate you are consuming, you may end up with ketones in your urine (see Of Ketones and Ketostix). Drinking enough water will help keep those ketones out of your urine by facilitating digestion.

Water may not literally help lower blood glucose levels, but it sets the stage for healthy, efficient digestion and general metabolism, which does facilitate the work your insulin supply faces at mealtime and snack time. So, for your health's sake, drink up, and "Lachiam." By the way, drinking water is also good for your skin. So how can you lose? You'll be beautiful on the inside and the outside—and all due to a simple, clear liquid that is not a drug and has no food value or calories. People use the word *miracle* all too freely these days, but water is truly a miracle.

dressing, and you're done. I dispensed with fresh vegetables when the washing and chopping was just too much for my busy schedule—not for my son, of course. He always had raw carrots or steamed broccoli, his favorites. By now, I was sick of broccoli and could hardly swallow it. I still took my vitamins, thank goodness.

I will say that I never abandoned red peppers, which someone had told me could help the pancreas. I'm not sure exactly how. Maybe the pancreas likes red. But, in any case, red peppers are rich in vitamin C and good for you all around, so they couldn't hurt.

AT 6 MONTHS

At this point, I began seeing a diabetologist who was closer to home and recommended by Dr. Richard Bernstein, my doctor at the time. The guru had done his work, and we both thought I could manage without the long trips to Mamaronak. Of course, if I had a problem, I wouldn't hesitate to call him. In addition, my internist felt my diet was a little extreme and wanted me to get another opinion.

My first appointment was illuminating. My mg/dL was 95. Great. But the nurse came back to tell me there were ketones (or acetone) in my urine. My doctor was worried about this and prescribed Ketostix for me to check my urine daily for ketones. When ketones appear in the urine, it can mean that a diabetic may be verging on ketoacidosis (see Insulin Reactions; and Ketoacidosis) or that you are not consuming a great deal of carbohydrates and your body has begun to utilize fat stores for energy, a byproduct of which is ketones. Coma is the end result of ketoacidosis.

Because I am a diabetic, my doctor wasn't willing to chalk it up to diet right away. He wanted me to add more carbohydrates to my daily fair and to test my urine every day. I wasn't on the verge of ketoacidosis, but I had plenty of ketones hanging around my urine. As my doctor said, "You can't defend yourself against a lion nearly as well when you're passed out." He was not worried about my blood sugar rising. He happily recommended whole grain bread, legumes, lentils, and low-sugar fruits. But I was worried. I was worried about everything, but then, I'm a worrier. I wasn't sure which I was worried more about—the possibility of coma or the possibility that my blood sugars might skyrocket when I added those sneaky carbs to my diet. I'd mourned the loss of beans and cantaloupe, and now I was equally terrified to take them back. Call me the jilted lover of the dietary set. Nevertheless, I took his advice to heart. This first visit was also when he told me to have my internist give me a blood test (this to save me money, since my internist takes my managed care plan but my diabetologist does not) that would determine if any cells of the pancreas had been destroyed, which would answer, once and for all, the question of whether or not I was a Type I diabetic.

Here I was again—on the rat race of the right diet, the right treatment plan, the right diagnosis. Home I went, to buy a loaf of seven grain bread and some cans of black beans and kidney beans, some lentils, an onion, and a red pepper. Bean salad, lentil salad, and bread—here I come. I wasn't overcome with joy, but I was more pleased than I'd like to admit about the prospect of a bean salad.

Being a typical product of our society, I must confess, I was also concerned about gaining weight, though not as concerned as I was about passing out in front of my son. So, terrified, I began. I snacked on almonds and walnuts. I ate a half a piece of a great multigrain bread, every day. I was glad to be back in the saddle. I stuck with my protein breakfast, on the theory that it was still a good idea to get my system started with as little carbohydrate as possible. I realized in my "fast and loose" period that I had been sloughing off when it came to drinking water (good for flushing ketones out of the system), and so I went back to flooding my system with H_2O.

Now, for the test. How was my urine? How was my blood sugar? The Ketostix showed a pale pink—a little more than a trace, but a lot less than had been registered at the doctor's office, which had been moderate to large (between mauve and plum colored on the stick). Okay, so I wasn't going to go into a coma. But how about the blood sugar? If that went through the roof, I'd end up running the risk of coma anyway. Not today, not tomorrow, but someday, and for the rest of my life. Not really, but I would be back to square one—facing insulin or oral agents. My blood sugar, however, stayed in the normal range. It was a little higher, 100–110, but I would take it. Over the next few weeks, I did gain 2 or 3 pounds, but I decided this was the least of my worries.

My internist gave me the blood test for eyelet cell damage (medical term tk), and the good news was that my pancreas was not damaged. As definitively as a diabetes diagnosis can be made, I was now considered a Type II diabetic. But who knows? There's always next year. My ketones were down to a trace— good enough for the doc. And I had my cantaloupe and strawberries back.

AFTER 1 YEAR

I am a much healthier person than I was before I was diagnosed with diabetes or than I was during my first year as a diabetic. I am also a much better diabetic than I was during that first year. I still eat a high-protein, low-carbohydrate diet, but as my body's needs change, I modify my daily plan. For example, if I see that my bgls are running a little high consistently, I'll hold back on my various whole grain breads and legumes. (To be honest, if I'm feeling a pound or two above my happiness level,

I'll do this too. Believe me it works. Off they go.). If my blood sugar is consistently on the low side of normal, I'll enjoy more of the company of my favorite carbohydrates.

This may or may not be medically accurate, but fairly well-trusted theory has it that there is a cumulative effect to lowering insulin resistance (therefore blood sugar). Over a period of months, your levels get better, even if you don't change a thing in your diet, simply because the system is now running more efficiently. From my personal evidence, I believe this. I still never eat sweets, but I've had a French fry off my son's plate, an order of fried calamari (fried in cornmeal), and an almond butter sandwich here and there with no significant modulation in my blood glucose levels.

I now eat a relatively healthy diet on all fronts every day. And I drink plenty of water. Here are some reasonable changes I made after a year in boot camp:

- I'm avoiding saturated fat more strictly. I put half and half in my coffee, sometimes, but that's it.
- I concentrate on getting enough omega-3, the good fat, from walnuts, fatty fish, and so on.
- I include vitamin-rich fruits in my diet every day, in small quantities.
- I eat fresh beets once in a while, even though they're high in sugar, because they're so good for you.

My percentages are as follows (remember that these are all approximations, since I can't live life any other way):

35 to 40 percent protein
30 to 35 percent fat
35 percent carbohydrate

THE FUNNEL APPROACH

Let me say at the outset that the following has no scientific validity, and I am not claiming that it does. But it works for me and my blood glucose levels, and that's the goal for each of us. In terms of when I consume my carbohydrates, I look at my dietary day as an inverted funnel.

Take breakfast as the narrowest part of the funnel. This means I consume almost no carbohydrates in the morning, except the minimal amount in my eggs or cottages cheese and the tiny bit of cream in my coffee. My morning snack comes to not much more than that, say 5 percent if I have a bran crisp and a slice of cheese. At lunch, the funnel widens. If I have a salad with dressing or a vegetable with a dipping sauce, I'm at approximately 10 percent. In the afternoon, if I've had the bran cracker in the morning, I'll have a zucchini "roll-up" to save my remaining carbs for dinner. Then at dinner, I can go wild. This is the widest part of the funnel. I enjoy a vegetable with hollandaise, a small portion of a bean salad or a half a slice of whole grain bread, and my glass of wine, which comes to between 15 and 20 percent, leaving my daily total right at about 35 percent, the ballpark area I shoot for now.

13

Recipes, Tricks, and Tips

I'LL TAKE MINE RAW: CRUCIFEROUS VEGETABLES, BETA CAROTENE, VITAMINS, AND YOU

I've never met a raw vegetable I didn't like better than a cooked vegetable. It's taken me a great deal of time to be able to say this and mean it, but I can say it now, and I do mean it, for a lot of reasons.

First of all, raw vegetables contain more vitamins and nutrients than cooked vegetables do, and that will never change. The longer you cook a vegetable, the less it has to give you in every way. In addition, you can eat about 1 cup of a low-carb vegetable, but you can eat as much as you want of that same vegetable raw. This means raw vegetables are great to snack on because you can't possibly eat too much.

Second, at the same time that boiling vegetables or overcooking them in other ways takes the starch out of them flavorwise, it also puts the starch into them. By this I mean, overcooking a vegetable breaks down its fiber content and turns it into a carbohydrate that is less complex than simple and replete in glucose that must be immediately assimilated.

If you do cook your vegetables, and we all do for family dinners and dinner parties—after all, crudité is crudité, not a course on the dinner plate—steaming is the best method. And I would say, except in extenuating circumstance, the only way.

To begin to incorporate raw vegetables into your daily dietary life, try serving them with a low-fat dip before dinner, whether you have guests or not. This is a perfect nosh for you, and who knows? You may end up improving the dietary habits of other members of your family purely by example.

Raw vegetables of choice include all peppers—green, red, orange, and yellow—broccoli, pea pods, endive, green beans, cabbage (in strips), and cauliflower, if you can stand it. Blanching asparagus for 1 minute can give it a fairly honorable place on this list too. I like raw asparagus, but I would not recommend it to everyone. So, a little blanch here and a little blanch there can help your appetite without destroying the nutrient and fiber content of your now favorite vegetables.

By the way, if keeping fresh vegetables available in the fridge is impossible for you on a daily basis, it should be noted that fresh frozen vegetables are just as good. In fact, in some cases, when the vegetables on sale aren't really fresh, "fresh frozen" may be the better choice.

Vegetable Tip

Tired of washing those veggies? Don't want to de-seed a red pepper and chop it up, either? You think it would be easier just to open a bag of chips for a snack? Well, try this. When you buy your fresh vegetables—every 3 days or so—take 10 minutes when you get home to wash and chop a selection of peppers, broccoli, and so forth. Then store them in your favorite Tupperware container, and you've got them at your fingertips whenever you want them, as convenient as that bag of chips and a far, far better thing to eat. If even this seems like too much work, many stores sell already chopped vegetables in small packages. They're a little bit more costly, but if you're having trouble getting on the vegetable wagon, it's worth the investment. You may also want to concentrate on vegetables that take less preparation, such as endive leaves—chop off the end of the endive and voilà, finger food—and snow pea pods.

EATING WITH THE FAMILY

So, your family is in rebellion. They won't eat what you want to eat. This is not an excuse to give up; it's a challenge. Yes, you can create an intricate food harmony at the dinner table without too much strain on your time, sanity, or pocketbook. And after all, if you have toddlers or teenagers, you're probably already used to a wide variety of mealtime choices. In many families, a catch-as-catch-can existence is already the order of the day. If this is true in your home, for once you're in luck. Besides, these days almost everyone is on a special diet, a restricted diet, or a life-enhancing diet of one kind or another, so it's probably as good a time as ever to declare that you have a diet of your own.

Variety In the Spice Rack

Spices are one of the true wonders of cooking. A single spice can change a dish from something plain and predictable to a new taste sensation. Here are my favorites:

- Basil
- Cilantro (Keep fresh cilantro in your crisper whenever possible.)
- Cinnamon (check the label to make sure no sugar has been added.)
- Cumin
- Garlic[*] (fresh or powdered)
- Ginger (fresh or powdered)
- Marjoram
- Nutmeg
- Onion (If you use fresh onions, use them raw in salads or sauté them very lightly. Cooked onions can be high in carbohydrates.)
- Oregano
- Parsley (Keep fresh parsley in your crisper whenever possible.)
- Rosemary
- Thyme

[*]An Ode to Garlic: Garlic is great, or as Les Blank put it in the title of his elegant movie, "Garlic Is as Good as Ten Mothers." This may be an overstatement, but not by much. Garlic can turn a plain piece of chicken into a feast or the same old salad into a tangy treat. Garlic enhances everything from fish, poultry, and meat to vegetables and salads. And it is indisputable across the board— from purveyors of alternative medicine to the medical community itself—that garlic is good for you. Fresh garlic, however, will contribute some carbohydrate grams to your day's total, but I think it's worth it. A teaspoon of crushed or minced garlic contains 2 grams of carbohydrate. Garlic powders run about 2 grams per teaspoon, and garlic salt (Lawry's Spice Blends) contains only .8 grams per teaspoon. Though nothing replaces the tang of fresh garlic, garlic powders and salts can add flavor.

If you have carbohydrate craving children, and you are not ready to wean them of this vice, there are alternatives to torturing yourself by making a big plate of white rice every night.

Here are some of them:
- If you have toddlers who will eat nothing but will inhale pasta with butter or parmesan, make a big pot of pasta at the beginning of the week, store it in the fridge in Tupperware, and dole it out on demand.
- Keep whole wheat muffins on hand and make "home-made" pizzas in the toaster oven—just add a little pre-shredded mozzarella to a split muffin and toast.
- Make main courses separately that can be used as toppings for pasta. Cook pasta separately. Combine the pasta and the main course at the table, or have *them* do it themselves.
- Use whole wheat or artichoke pasta, just in case you nibble.
- Keep a cabinet filled with different kinds of rice cakes and crackers for "carb munchies."
- Keep whole grain bread in the freezer and use bread and butter as your carb course. Kids love to use a butter knife to butter it themselves, and it teaches manual dexterity.
- Keep baking potatoes in the house. You won't eat them, but they're an easy addition to any meal, as long as you remember to turn on the oven and then take them out 45 or so minutes later (or much less in the microwave).
- Order out, when you just can't face it. Protein for you and them. Starch for them alone.
- Slowly but surely convert the family to the whole grain way of life.

TEN-MINUTE MEALS

There is probably no such thing as a ten-minute meal, unless it's a Big Mac, and then you've already spent ten minutes in line (and you can't eat it anyway). But there are ways of getting close, without jeopardizing your blood glucose levels.

If you're an airline pilot or flight attendant, a short order cook, a television actor, an assembly line worker, a newscaster, a school teacher, a politician stumping for re-election, a circus performer, a rock 'n' roll musician on tour, a nurse or doctor, a mental health care worker, a traveling wildlife veterinarian, a professional baseball player or sports columnist, a member of the ice capades, or if you have any other impossible job, you probably put food last on your day's agenda, that is, except to get some of it into you at some time. Rest assured that you can do this and still lower your blood glucose levels. Here's how.

Keep the following on hand at home:

- Keep canned tuna, canned beans, olives, artichoke hearts, hearts of palm, capers, and any other low-carb taste treat that you like on hand all the time.
- Keep fresh frozen vegetables in the freezer.
- Keep your meat of choice in the freezer. Put it in the fridge in the morning to thaw.
- Keep low-carb bran crackers on hand.
- Keep low-carb cheeses on hand.
- Keep cold cuts on hand.
- If you don't have a microwave, get one to heat your pre-cooked meals.
- For a fast, fast meal as you steam a great mess'o broccoli or your vegetable of choice, heat up a cracker sandwich with ham and cheese in the microwave.
- Prepare meals in advance on your day off, and store them in fridge or freezer, particularly if you have a family.

- If you have a family and you feel overwhelmed some evening, ask them to fend for themselves or ask your spouse to cook. Or, they can order out, and you can make your ten-minute meal. All of you still can sit down together. Worse things have happened. Worse things could happen, like you eating the pizza they ordered because you got too hungry. Don't do it.

Here are some tips for when you're on the road:
- If you must order the Big Mac, discard the bun before it tempts you, add mayo to the beef patty, and enjoy it with extra lettuce (they will give it to you).
- If you are flying, call ahead for a special meal. Say you're diabetic or just say you have extensive allergies or say you keep kosher. The kosher meal is still better than the regular meal for diabetics.
- In restaurants, declare you need special attention before you begin to order. The waitperson will always be more sympathetic if he or she realizes you "need" to be "picky," rather than that you are just picky. (If you don't like picky, use particular.)
- Travel with a jar of walnuts or almonds.
- Wherever you end up, in whatever town, shop for cheese (cheese sticks are easy because they come prewrapped) and other low-carb, non-spoiling foods, and keep them in your room.

CONDIMENT MAGIC

In the best sense of the word, a good condiment can be the bribe that leads you to eat a healthy food you might have avoided. For example, if you add a little mustard and low-fat mayo together, you have a dip into which you can dip your not-yet-favorite raw vegetable, then eat it and learn to love it, with a little help from your friends, in this case, condiments.

Here are some great condiments I have known:

- Mayonnaise and low-fat mayonnaise: Actually there are now "lite" and low-fat mayonnaise on the market. I go for the Hellmann's low-fat, which has the lowest carb content and is also lower in calories, since, of course, fewer of those calories are from fat.
- Mustard: From simple to complex, Grey Poupon, Pommery, "moutarde de meaux," and tarragon mustard top my list. (Check the label to make sure there is no sugar added.)
- Capers: Capers cheer up tuna salad, chicken salad, a niçoise dish (make it a salad, not a pasta, or leave the pasta sidedish optional for guests).
- Olives: Not too many, but a few pitted black olives crumbled in a salad can make you feel like you are not being deprived.
- Low-sodium soy sauce
- Horseradish
- Garlic powder

The condiment caveat is that many condiments (and seasonings) are remarkably high in sodium. Not to complicate your life too much, but as you tend your diabetes, so you must tend your other risk factors—such as that for heart disease, which rises as you get older—and this means being a salty dog without eating too much salt. So check the labels. Choose garlic powder over garlic salt, choose low-sodium products whenever possible, and avoid things like A-1 Sauce and other high-sodium seasonings. You'll see from the labels that they're way over the top—say 1,000 mg.

ORGANIC FOODS

Organic foods will not lower your blood sugar as far as I can tell, but they have once again become a possibility in life. It is probably a good idea to embrace foods that are not high in preservatives and additives. Why not? However, don't forget that many organic farms are not up to the hygienic standards you might want to embrace.

I try to use organic products in the foods and substances we partake of every day. That means that I use organic coffees for myself (mostly decaf) and organic eggs (which tend to be higher in omega-3 fatty acids, the right kind). I also serve organic milk to my son and organic half and half to myself. Vegetables and fruits are mostly organic—but washed extremely well. And I make no claim to partaking only of organic produce.

Like everything else, be careful. Shop at a reputable health food store. Make sure all produce is fresh. Be particularly careful about purchasing organic meat and fish. Make sure the products you purchase are fresh and that you trust the source.

And if, for whatever reason, you don't want to go to a health food store, you can still manage your diabetes very well. By the way, the sweets you buy there are still, for the most part, off limits for you: Health food/organic substances do not equal dessert substitutes.

A Note on Organic Foods

I have a friend who says a little bit of pesticide will help you build up immunity. She says this with pesticide in cheek, but goodness knows, there are crazier dietary theories these days. I don't agree with her, even in jest, yet nor do I think that we are doomed to an early end by pesticides. That notwithstanding, I do have a young son, and it can't hurt to do the best you can by nutrition, for yourself as well as the kid. Therefore, I've come up with my own theory (which I've stated before): The foods we eat daily are mostly organic, such as eggs, the vegetables I buy, the juices for him, the coffee for me, and the milk and cream (but this is not always so). Since we're so into percentages, I would say we're about 40 to 50 percent organic. Whether or not you agree with this approach, there are a few things you should know.

Fruits and vegetables considered organic have been grown without the use of any pesticides in the soil. And livestock is considered organic if it has been fed only organic food products. Both the United States Department of Agriculture (USDA) and the Food and Drug Administration (FDA) consider that by their standards, the levels of pesticides in the foods we eat are acceptable. You may or may not agree with this. My one caveat is that these levels are assessed by estimating the average amount of fresh produce consumed by Americans and calculating the amount of pesticides in such portions. Methinks Americans are eating more fresh fruits and vegetables than the conservative estimates of institutions—at least we diabetics are eating those vegetables. (The FDA estimates include only small portions of fruits and vegetables.)

So if you can and if you care, you might want to devote at least a portion of your daily fair to organic products. Remember, though, that organic products, like everything else, are not perfect. Check, first of all, to make sure all organic milk is pasteurized, for the safety of you and your children. Unpasteurized milk can be more dangerous than a residue of pesticide. Also, buy your organic produce, meat, and poultry from a merchant you've come to trust. From farm to farm, the definition of organic changes. Make sure that for you it's a definition you can trust.

And don't forget that we're at much higher risk of health problems from tobacco, alcohol, drug addiction, obesity, you name it, than we are from pesticides.

ALCOHOL

As the aunt of my sister-in-law's mother once said, "Too much is not good." This goes for just about everything, particularly when you are diabetic, and it is never more true than when the subject is alcohol.

Whether you are diabetic or not, continued alcohol abuse can and will damage not only your liver but also every organ in your body. Your heart suffers. Your brain suffers. Even your skin suffers. After years of heavy drinking, the liver becomes damaged and unable to adequately process and store fat. So if you are a heavy drinker and find that even with the added inspiration of trying to manage your diabetes through diet that you still can't cut back on your drinking, you should seek help. There are more and more programs that deal successfully with alcoholism.

All of this said, now for the good news. If you like wine and do not have a drinking problem, you should be delighted to know that wine, red wine in particular, should become part of your program. A small amount of wine daily in not simply neutral to your goal but helpful. Not only does it protect your heart, but it also aids digestion. Some recent studies have shown that particularly red wine may increase insulin sensitivity in the body—good news for diabetics who like their wine. In fact, this is probably the reason why wine aids digestion.

Good News

Attention. More good news for diabetics. A recent study has shown that moderate consumption of alcoholic beverages is as good for diabetics as it is for other adults. Drinking one to two drinks per day was found to lower cholesterol in diabetics, while having no deleterious effects on blood sugar levels. (Remember, no sweet, sugary mixed drinks, though.) So, you can go ahead and sip your wine or order that special martini without guilt or negative consequences as long as your alcohol consumption remains moderate.

Isn't it interesting just how much insulin has to do with everything? Thanks, in part, to the work of Drs. Michael and Mary Dan Eades, we are beginning to understand the paramount role insulin plays in maintaining overall health.

When you add wine to the program, of course, you'll add a moderate amount. That means between one and two glasses per day. (Women should try to keep it to one glass a day, in general, since studies have shown that women are more sensitive to the effects of alcohol than men.) The carbohydrate value of a dry red or white wine is approximately 1 to 1.5 grams per ounce. Remember to count the wine in your carbohydrate allotment, and stay away from beer, which is higher in carbohydrate value, and distilled spirits (though their carbohydrate value is virtually nil—remember it's distilled alcohol—there is evidence that distilled spirits can decrease insulin sensitivity). However, if you treat yourself to a martini a month, this will not occur. So eat, drink wine, increase your insulin sensitivity, and lower your blood glucose levels. Then, be merry.

A Snacking Strategy

If you play your snack cards right, snacks can be your ally in your new regime, not your enemy. The best way to do this is to give yourself as little opportunity as possible to veer off course. In other words, keep "safe snacks" in plentiful supply at home and ban the other kind, those nasty, high-carb snacks, from your home.

Here are a few snack possibilities (some are more portable than others):

- A slice of ham (1 oz.) on a bran cracker
- A piece of cheese (1 oz.) on a bran cracker
- A green salad with oil and vinegar or a low-carbohydrate dressing
- Broccoli (1/5) or other low-carbohydrate vegetable with a low-carb dip
- One hard-boiled egg with salt
- One-egg "egg salad" made with a tablespoon of mayonnaise
- Cottage cheese (1/4 to 1/2 cup, depending on your carb allotment during the day)
- Walnuts or other low-carbohydrate nuts (1 oz.)

CAFFEINE

No doubt about it, caffeine is a drug, and, of course, this is both its asset and its liability. So, go for it, but go for it in moderation. And that word *moderation*—if you hate it, you're going to have to learn to love it. How caffeine affects each of us varies, but for most of us, one or two cups acts almost immediately as a stimulus. Stimulation can help exacerbate stress levels—which is not good for us diabetics. In addition, caffeine also stimulates the kidneys, which then leads to the increased production of urine. Once again, that's not what we need. This means, you certainly cannot count your caffeinated beverage among the eight glasses of water that you need to drink per day. A cup or two of coffee will not hurt you or raise your blood sugar level, and during the first weeks of this regimen, it may even help eliminate feelings of fatigue that may plague you. But large quantities of caffeine often lead to restlessness, insomnia, and trembling, as well as gastrointestinal problems including diarrhea—which can cause dehydration, which is, once again, not good

A Sandwich by Any Other Name

While the Earl of Sandwich might be turning over in his grave, two pieces of bread do not necessarily a sandwich make. It's true that one of the things you might love and probably will be eating less of will be that good old American standby, the sandwich. Portable, edible anywhere, and a very creative format for an entire meal, your basic, white-bread sandwich is basically off limits forevermore.

Don't despair, however, there are alternatives to the classic sandwich. They include the cracker sandwich, the whole-grain-half, and the messy plate sandwich:

• *The Cracker Sandwich:* You might resist the chewing quotient, at first, but you can enjoy a perfectly good, perfectly portable ham and cheese on rye cracker instead of rye bread. Just place your ham, low-fat cheese, and low-fat mayo between two crunchy whole grain rye crackers, and you're on your way to a quick and easy lunch that won't overload you with carbohydrates.

• *The Whole-Grain-Half:* If you want to use some of your daily carb allotment, use one piece of whole grain bread and make an open-faced sandwich. Add your favorite lettuce,

for us diabetics. So if you are drinking more than three cups of coffee a day, you should cut back.

SALT

If you have no complications resulting from diabetes, your blood pressure is normal, and your circulation is normal, salt is basically a neutral component in your diet. However, most Americans eat too much salt in general, so it's a good idea to watch your salt intake anyway. Too much salt does nobody any good.

RECIPES

This is not a cookbook or a book of recipes. God knows there are enough of those—for every occasion, every budget, every ailment, and every ethnic group and/or cultural persuasion, and more. This is a book for diabetics, one that will give you no

whether it be mache and field greens or iceberg (try to avoid the iceberg, but if it's your greatest love, indulge), load on the tuna or chicken salad, the ham and the cheese, or even last night's steak, and enjoy your sandwich with half the carbohydrates.

- *The Messy Plate Sandwich:* If you order a sandwich in a restaurant, never be afraid to make a mess. Go ahead, be an inventor. Take one piece off the top of each half sandwich and combine what's left. You'll get to chew on more and skip a whole bread slice worth of carbohydrates. If you are in a restaurant on business and it specializes in sandwiches only, order one of those trendy sandwiches—you know, rare tuna with daicon strips, or chicken with bacon, chipotle sauce, and who knows what—and just remove the bread and eat the fillings. If anyone questions you, just say, "Haven't you heard? Carbs are out." And don't be embarrassed. People admire someone who doesn't "clear his or her plate." It means they're concentrating on other things, like the business at hand perhaps.

excuses not to do better by yourself and not to keep your disease under control or at least within manageable parameters.

Once you learn the carbohydrate values of foods and the substitutions that can be made in cooking everything from main courses to desserts, you'll find that you will be able to navigate your favorite recipes by making intelligent substitutions as you go. For further recipes, you might try *Protein Power* by Drs. Michael and Mary Dan Eades, though you will have to adjust the carbohydrate content of some, since it will be higher than your allotment in most cases. You may also consult *Dr. Richard Bernstein's Diabetes Solution*. His recipes may be particularly helpful as you begin; then they may drive you crazy. Once you begin to normalize blood sugar, however, they may be unnecessarily restrictive regarding carbohydrates. Once again, remember to let your Glucometer be your guide.

You have no excuse to eat poorly. Shopping, cooking, serving, eating well, and saving food have never been easier or more practically outlined by experts.

Zucchini Roll-Ups (or Any Fresh Vegetable and Protein, for That Matter)

Fear not, there is life after bread and finger food after bread. And you will feel more like a creative resourceful person after you have read this section and applied it to your life.

I can't say I wept when I realized the sandwich, as I knew it, was a thing of the past for me. All that simplicity, all that practicality, all that portability, all that time saving, gone like a dandelion to seed on a windy day. But, of course, this is not so. Not to sound like an old rock song about love for the moment, but all you need for a sandwich is something to hold onto. And not to sound like a jaded X-generation song about getting whatever it is for the moment, but all you need for an hors d'oeuvre is something to pick up.

TUNA SALAD, CANNELLINI STYLE

So, tuna salad is dull. But it is nutritional, and it is easy. And life without a can of tuna fish in the cupboard is not acceptable.

When that can is all you have and you're hungry and you're about to bolt to the supermarket for ice cream—not a reasonable alternative—think about the following (I'm not saying you'll make this choice the first time, but you might make it the second time).

Mix a can of cannellini beans with a can of tuna fish, add a pinch of basil, garlic salt, and/or Crazy Salt, a teaspoon of red wine vinegar or balsamic vinegar, and a tablespoon or more of olive oil. If you have a lemon, squeeze a quarter on the whole "shmeer." Then toss. Place the salad on a crisp lettuce leaf or two, and serve it with a half slice of whole grain bread.

SHRIMP SALAD NIÇOISE

Just to keep my salad days interesting, I sometimes substitute shrimp for tuna and add other interesting ingredients to what is basically a niçoise-type salad. To prepare a niçoise-type salad, add eggs, olives, and fresh green beans (no tomatoes); use some field greens and bean sprouts for your "base," so to speak. Then substitute your protein source: rock shrimp, regular shrimp, or even cooked chicken breasts. Mix a dressing of mayo, oil and vinegar, and mustard to taste, and you'll have a new and appetizing salad.

MANY BEAN, MANY PEPPER SALAD, PLUS ONION AND GARLIC

Beans are great, and they only cause the stereotypical havoc to your digestive system, if you're not used to them. If you eat beans regularly, they won't bother you at all. So, get in the habit.

Peppers are great in every way. They're an important cruciferous vegetable. They're low in carbohydrate. And there's at least a rumor that they work well to restore the potency of the pancreas. (Remember that this is a rumor spread by friends of alternative medicine. I just thought it couldn't hurt to mention it, since peppers are worth including in your diet whether or not this little fillip of good is true.)

So here's what I do: I toss a can of black beans and cannellini beans together. Then I chop a red pepper, a yellow pepper, and a green pepper—and add. (Or chop up whatever peppers are available in your area. I recently found white peppers, which made a nice contrast that Martha Stewart might have been proud of.) Add one chopped red onion and one chopped garlic clove. Toss well with virgin olive oil (and a little flaxseed oil) and balsamic vinegar or the vinegar of your choice. Mix well. Add parsley and your herbs of choice, and Crazy Salt and pepper, if you like. Toss again.

DESSERTS, IF YOU MUST

Soy milk and soybean flour can be substituted in some of your favorite dessert recipes, as can Equal tablets or saccharine or Stevia for the sweetener. Eggs, cream, butter, and even milk are on your list, though you might want to substitute half and half for milk to keep the carb content down. Try a cheesecake recipe to start. For the crust, substitute crumbled bran crackers or another low-carbohydrate cracker for graham crackers. See what you think and see what it does to your blood sugar. Don't ever make yourself a pear tart. Your blood sugar will know.

You may also eat any sugar-free Jell-O or Jell-O pudding. You may also want to try your favorite cheese and nuts instead of something sweet to finish the meal. You can also make frozen "pops" with your favorite diet soda, if this appeals. Make sure your soda doesn't contain the *g* word (glucose) or the suffix "-ose." (Don't buy pops at the store. They're fruit pops, and they're loaded with sugar.) Eventually, as your blood sugars stabilize, you can have a serving of cantaloupe or strawberries with whipped cream flavored with your favorite flavor extract. The possibilities aren't endless, but there are possibilities.

FOOD TRICKS

DIP ONE, EAT TWO

Make an easy dip by mixing 1 teaspoon of your favorite mustard or salsa with approximately 1 cup of low-fat mayonnaise. Then get your crudités ready—raw broccoli, cauliflower, red pepper, and green beans are good choices. When you dip, dip half the vegetable in. Then do it again with another great raw vegetable. This way you up your ante without double-dipping into fat and calorie problems you don't need.

SIX ALMOND MONTE

Nuts do have calories, but let's not hold this against the almond—an almost perfect food. Almonds contain the "right" kind of fat, omega-3 fatty acids. They contain protein, and they are metabolized more slowly than other carbohydrates. Three tablespoons of almonds (a lot more than I'm suggesting you eat at one sitting) contain 15 grams of fat, but only 1 gram is from saturated fat. So you're safe there. The total carbohydrate count for the same amount is only 6 grams, and while not super high in fiber, this portion size roles in at 3 grams of fiber—not bad. And we all know fiber is good for what ails us. You also get 6 grams of protein for your portion size. All in all, an almond is a perfect, little fuel morsel, except for one thing—the calorie content for this size snack is 180, and 130 of those calories are from fat. I'm not particularly worried about the fat, since the fat is your friend. But that's a lot of calories—and one more reason to keep your nut snacks squirrel-sized and not elephant-sized. Almonds are also bite-sized, portable, and very tasty, and they give you something you can really chew on. All of this makes them an excellent snack investment, as long as you exercise some control. Pick a number, your favorite number between five and ten, and make this your almond allotment. Pack this snack ration in a plastic baggy in your purse or pocket to chomp on when you're on the go and getting too hungry to curb your wish list of "no-nos." Or eat your almonds just before lunch or dinner or going out to stave off the major hunger pangs that could cause you to overeat and thus go into carbohydrate overload.

I'm a big fan of walnuts, too. They're even higher in fat than almonds, but most of it is the "good" fat, or omega-3 fatty acid.

Using Decaf Coffee as a Useful Crutch

If you're feeling deprived, have a cup of decaf coffee with cream with your morning or afternoon snack. Of course, you don't have to eliminate caffeine from your diet, but you do want to avoid having too much. You can count decaf with cream as a "free" treat, and you can have more than one cup. A few cups in the afternoon may help you through the first week or two, during the time when almost everything that has to do with your diet will feel anywhere from a little to very restrictive.

Flavor-Full, Keeps the Cravings Away

For a taste treat, use flavor extracts to sweeten your coffee (with cream) or your yogurt. Or use a flavor extract in a glass of seltzer to make a refreshing "cocktail."

Not So Mock Hollandaise

Hollandaise sauce is high in saturated fat, without a doubt, but the carbohydrate content is nil, and it's not hard to make. As you enter the virtuous world of vegetables, you may feel less than excited by your nutritious and cruciferous leafy greens, dark greens, yellows et al. A tablespoon of hollandaise can turn a duty into a treat, making asparagus, broccoli, cauliflower, or green beans into the most appetizing thing on the menu.

KEEP YOUR FREEZER FULL AND YOUR CRISPER DRY

As it was once said of Mt. Everest, so it can be said of that sole piece of chocolate cake in an otherwise naked ice box: "Because it was there." To avoid the blood sugar curdling consequences of such a blatant rationalization, avoid temptation by keeping tempting but healthy alternatives within easy reach.

In your freezer, you should always have some frozen, low-fat protein in stock, such as boneless, skinless chicken breasts or your favorite cut of low-fat meat, as well as low-fat breakfast sausages, if that appeals to you in the morning. Your freezer should also contain an assortment of fresh frozen vegetables to choose from at dinnertime, after a hectic day.

Ideally, your crisper should be filled with fresh vegetables and salad greens. But this is not a perfect world, and so a cornucopia of nature's best may not always greet you when you open that crisper drawer. At worst, you may find yourself facing heads of soggy lettuce and a limp zucchini. At this point, it's time to practice the 2-foot toss into the garbage can, mop out that crisper, and shop again. A 5-day-old vegetable isn't worth the time it takes you to chew it. Try to stock up on fresh produce every few days and vary what you buy to keep your choices interesting. And don't let anything languish in that crisper long enough to wilt and start to make its own puree in the bottom of the drawer.

Here's what you should have in your fridge as much of the time as possible: cold cuts, cheeses (I still say low fat, unless you're really skinny), including string cheese sticks, which are easy to grab and munch, low-carbohydrate dips and sauces to keep those vegetables interesting, cream for your coffee, plain yogurt (low-fat yogurts have more carbohydrates than regular yogurt, so buy regular), and soy milk. You may also want to keep No-Cal syrups on hand as sweeteners for those yogurts or for a soy milk milk shake. Keep some prepared sugar-free Jell-O on hand to help manage your sweet tooth. There should be a dozen eggs (preferably organic, which tend to by higher in omega-3 fatty acid). There might also be a Tupperware container filled with hard-boiled eggs for quick snacks or an impromptu egg salad. On your side shelf, you'll want to have your mayo, mustard, horseradish, capers, and a jar of minced garlic on hand, just to keep your gustatory life interesting.

Don't hoard leftovers. They tend to lose their nutritional value very quickly. Keep them for a day or two at the most. And don't bring "doggy bags" home from restaurants you may be tempted to save foods that you shouldn't have ordered in the first place—like dessert. In addition, if sweets do find their way into your home for birthday or anniversary celebrations, for example, don't save the leftovers. Toss the cake and protect yourself. Those in the house who want them will always get enough sweets. It is not your job to torture yourself in order to provide for them. You've got enough on your plate without cake.

Have Tupperware, Will Travel

Never underestimate the importance of containers. They make life easier by getting leftovers out of the way without a lot of plastic wrap or aluminum foil or other forms of red tape, so to speak. They also come in all shapes and sizes, custom tailored to storing anything from that last piece of roast beef to the leftover asparagus for tomorrow. Dips and sauces can also be stored for future use, giving you no excuses to indulge in unhealthy snacks.

Dipping into Dips

Shop around for dips, the perfect accompaniments for all your favorite fresh vegetables. These days the dip is no longer relegated to that homespun favorite, the classic onion soup dip. There's baba ghannoush, hummus, hummus with lemon, hummus with spinach, tahini with this, tahini with that, low-fat blue cheese dips, low-fat clam dips. And every day, profit conscious and enlightened companies (health food oriented or not) are creating new dips, including black bean dips, white bean hummus dips, and more. And that's only a short list. If you think you can't bear the thought of a raw vegetable, try an appetizing dip. You can make one at home, simply by mixing mayonnaise and tarragon mustard (provided you like mayonnaise). You can also mix blue cheese, cottage cheese, and a low-fat sour cream in the blender for a homemade dip that could help get those veggies into your mouth where they belong.

DINING TIPS

HOW TO BE A LOVING AND APPRECIATIVE GUEST WITHOUT RAISING YOUR BLOOD SUGAR

I was once marooned at a dinner party given by a friend who's a wonderful minister at a great church in Greenwich Village. I say marooned because he was making lasagna from scratch with homemade noodles. Homemade noodles—how could I insult a minister's homemade noodles. There were only four of us at dinner, so I could hardly lose myself in a crowd. The only hors d'oeuvre was chips and salsa—a big no-no. There was no cheese and certainly not any whole grain crackers, just bread. There was, however, a green salad in the making, and I offered to make the salad dressing, something I'm not too bad at. Devious me, I then asked if he had any Parmesan cheese in the fridge. I added it to the salad, telling him it was a taste trick I had learned over the years (which it is). If salad was to be my main course, at least I'd have the pleasure and the calories of a little Parmesan.

Looking back, I would have gone ahead and blown it and eaten the lasagna. As it was, I was new to the diabetic game, green you might say, and I was extremely worried about not following my regimen pretty much to the letter. I sipped my wine before I ate (to aid digestion) and did taste the lasagna. It was delicious, but I was afraid to have any more. I moved food around on my plate, picked out bites of cheese and ate them, and filled up on salad. No one was offended. Everything went smoothly. Of course, I skipped dessert. I'm still welcomed in my minister friend's fold. But then, he is a person of God in the true sense.

A JUG OF WINE, A PIECE OF CHEESE, NO LOAF, NOT THOU, BUT WHOLE GRAIN CRACKERS

Now, as a somewhat seasoned and mature diabetic, I do it differently. I don't go to that many formal dinner parties, but my son and I often have dinner with friends. When invited, I

Sweets for the Sweet Deprived

You say you're depressed, too depressed to say good-bye to your old pal "sugar," even though sugar was one of the gang of bad influences that got you to this pretty spot in the first place. So you say you're codependent . . . not even that . . . dependent. This plan, you say, is hopeless for you. Well stop. You can do it. And you can do it while still wrapping your tongue around sweet tastes.

Here are some staples for your sweet tooth cabinet:
- *No-Cal Brand Syrup:* No-Cal syrups truly do contain no carbohydrates and no calories. You could use one of the many flavors, such as chocolate, strawberry, or black cherry, to sweeten a plain yogurt.

- *Saccharine, Equal Tablets, Stevia:* These are the sugar substitutes that you can use without deleterious effects on your blood sugar and that can be substituted in baking or to flavor plain yogurt or a small portion of cottage cheese (see Chapter 13, Recipes, Tricks, and Tips).
- *Flavor Extracts:* The good news is that almost all flavor extracts, from vanilla to lemon, are safe for the diabetic. They don't raise blood sugar. So you can use them in your coffee, for an added treat with cream, to sweeten your seltzer into a "soda," or in baking.
- *Sugar Free Jell-O and Jell-O Puddings:* The Jell-O products

always ask what I can bring, and I bring what the hosts request, if they do. In addition to what they request or if they don't request a thing, I always bring an interesting cheese and a whole grain cracker, usually the Wasa brand—a little less austere than my bran crackers. The carb value of one slice is 8 grams or 3 percent of the total calories—a treat for me, and maybe a new taste for my friends. Actually, I've started somewhat of a trend downtown. The crackers I bring are then sought out. Friends call to ask where they can buy this cheese, that cracker. Oh, and by the way, I bring a bottle of wine, too. It's not that expensive. After all, I'm not cooking dinner at home. And just in case there isn't anything I can eat, I'm protected. In addition, of course, rather than being rude, I've been a generous guest.

However, most importantly, never eat anything to please someone else.

happen to be the best at doing what they preach, that is, providing a sugar-free dessert. They're an essential mainstay of any diabetic with a sweet tooth.

- *Soy Milk and Soybean Flour* (for substitutions in baking, see Chapter 13, Recipes, Tricks, and Tips): You can combine soy milk, ice, and your flavor extract of choice for an after-dinner (or after-lunch) "milk shake." Don't add it to a hot drink, however. It will curdle.
- *Low-Carbohydrate Crackers* (for substitutions in baking, see Chapter 13, Recipes, Tricks, and Tips).
- *Nuts:* Try having half an ounce to an ounce of your favorite nut with a low-carbohydrate cheese (that is, a hard cheese) for dessert with your last half-glass of wine.
- *Chewing Gum:* A sugar-free chewing gum may be all you need to sweeten your evening after dinner. Choose Trident or another brand that averages about 1 gram of carbohydrate per stick. Make sure to check labels for glucose or any other "-ose."
- *Whipped Cream:* Yes. You're not seeing things. Cream is low in carbohydrate. Whip it up with one of your acceptable sweeteners (Equal tablets, saccharine, or Stevia), flavor it with a No-Cal syrup and eat it alone, or use it as a topping on almost anything from Jell-O to yogurt to your morning coffee.

MANAGING YOUR DIABETES
WITH DIET, WITHOUT CREATING OTHER
HEALTH PROBLEMS

So great, you've got your blood sugar under control. But your cholesterol is raging. What good is that? Not much.

Those first few months of my low blood sugar regimen were clearly not giving me the hearty amounts of fruits and cruciferous vegetables that are now recommended for a cancer prevention diet. In addition, the lack of legumes and whole grains would have been unconscionable for those who tout the benefits of fiber (hence the Metamucil). And obviously in those first weeks, I might have seemed a candidate for scurvy had I not been taking my multivitamin and my vitamin C supplement.

While those 2 weeks might be considered a somewhat drastic dietary measure, I considered them a necessary investment—a crash course in normalizing blood glucose. And when you consider the contortions Americans often put themselves into when it comes to diet and food indulgences, my diet wasn't really all that bad. Besides, it worked. I would not recommend, however, staying on such a diet for a long period of time. If you can't keep blood glucose regulated when you add more vegetables and a moderate amount of whole grains and legumes, you should talk to your doctor about taking oral agents.

Here are some concerns you might have:
- *Your Cholesterol and Your Heart*: Interestingly enough, managing your insulin production and, therefore, blood glucose levels is also good for your heart. This dietary regimen should raise your "good" cholesterol level (HDL) while lowering or at least not raising your "bad" cholesterol level (LDL). So rather than increasing your risk of heart disease, your new regimen will protect your heart as well as control your diabetes.

- *Getting Enough Vitamins and Minerals*: You should be taking a multivitamin that provides you with adequate doses of all the B vitamins (in particular folic acid), as well as all your other vitamins and minerals. In addition, discuss with your doctor taking a potassium supplement, since most of our potassium comes from oranges, orange juice, and bananas, not your foods of choice right now.
- *Osteoporosis:* Your diet should provide you with more than enough calcium, but if you are a woman who is pregnant, going through menopause, or post-menopausal, your doctor may want you to take a calcium supplement.
- *Getting Enough Fiber:* Since fiber may be beneficial in regulating blood sugar, you don't want to stint here. Your raw or lightly steamed "fresh frozen" vegetables will provide you with lots of fiber, as will your bran and whole grain crackers. When you add on legumes and lentils as your blood glucose normalizes, you should be in excellent shape. Just in case, you may want to stick with a dose of Metamucil a day.

WHEN YOU NEED MORE HELP

Okay—so you've read every book, including this one, and you can't do it. This is not the time to toss in the towel, because—guess what—there is no towel. This is the time to admit to yourself that you need help, of which there is plenty.

If you find that after a month or two, I'll leave your level of desperation up to you, you cannot manage a new meal schedule and a nutrition plan that helps to control your blood glucose levels, first talk to your endocrinologist. Then think about the following. In many cities and medium-sized towns, there are caterers and food mavens. Why not make this convenience work for you?

I have a diabetic friend who was one of the first to "use" me as a diabetic hot line, if you will; he could not manage changing his diet either by himself or with his wife's help. Since they live in New York City, it was easy for me to help him, but it wasn't that easy. He wouldn't admit he had a problem with the food intake aspect for some time. He went on oral medication, instead. Then we started talking. (I am not a doctor. I don't play one on TV. But I've been through a lot.) Eventually, we discussed the notion of catered meals—not the expensive, not the big time, not the party animal kind of "catered." He had his meals (dinner and sometimes lunch) catered for a month. His blood glucose levels decreased substantially and normalized. In other words, they were not rising and falling, willy-nilly. He then went off his oral medication. He quit the caterer. (They were not rich.) But he took everything he learned from that month and put it into a durable program for managing diabetes. He's lost 10 pounds, and he hasn't been back on oral medications since.

This may or may not happen to you. But once again, I'm trying to tell you that you've got more control than you think. And if you feel out of control, there are a lot of ways that you can seek help. Remember, you've got the disease that can be managed.

If you really can't hack the diet, talk to your doctor about oral agents or insulin. Remember, the most important thing is controlling your blood glucose levels. Whatever method works for you is the one that you should choose. But don't forget that taking insulin or an oral agent is not an excuse to eat poorly and indulge in sweets. You're still going to have to be careful about what you eat. To boost your self-discipline, you may want to try the Weight Watchers program, a tried and true weight loss program that emphasizes changes in lifestyle, not just diet.

part 5

The Sisyphus Strategy: Lift Weights, Walk Uphill, Don't Stop

Sisyphus had his rock; I have my 7-year-old son's room. It's a bright room, filled with life, love, hard cover and paperback books, baseballs, Legos, action figures, magic markers, stuffed animals, drawings, games, videos, clothes, and these days, even homework assignments. It's the biggest room in our apartment, and it's where the fun is. It's also where the mess is, and I am always picking up. No matter how much I do, no matter how much my son helps, I find myself invariably bending and lifting, pushing that rock of order up that hill of chaos. The diligent Ms. Sisyphus, up, up, up, against the odds.

What does all of this have to do with diabetes? Not much, at least on the surface. But if you look more closely at Sisyphus and his rock and his doggedness, you'll begin to see a connection. It has to do with weight and resistance and resisting the impulse to quit.

As a diabetic, anaerobic exercise—exercise that depends on increased resistance and does not use oxygen—can be pretty close to your best friend. If you were to literally walk uphill, carrying free weights (in this case, as opposed to pushing a rock), you would be burning glucose—and the more glucose you burn, the less you tax your insulin supply. So while anaerobic exercise is work and, therefore, not a miracle, it's nice work for a diabetic, and you can get it.

And if being told again and again that exercise will help you manage your diabetes hasn't reached you, let me add this note from the American Heart Association (and please, take heed). Exercise can and does increase your longevity in all situations. A moderately active person is less likely to die of any cause— be it an accident, diabetes, heart disease, or cancer—than a sedentary person. And a highly active person is far less likely to die of any of the above causes. I don't know about you, but for me, this is as good as saying, "The gold is at Fort Knox."

In this section, you'll see how you can add physical activity to your life relatively painlessly and gain the benefits of anaerobic exercise while also maintaining cardiovascular health and your general flexibility and stamina.

14

Upping the Activity Ante in Your Daily Life

Here is the hard cheese. After drinking water—and presuming it is possible to consume a rudimentary number of calories per day—nothing is more important to maintaining the life of the body (and therefore the possibility of the life of the mind) than exercise. There is no way around it The body can even process white bread into something. This is not to say you should eat white bread. But all the body can do with a sedentary life is nothing. And nothing is worse than nothing. Stay still. Don't exercise. Don't move. Come up with excuses, good as they may be—the pain of arthritis, a heart condition, a busy life as a full time mother or father, wife or husband, computer programmer, executive, movie producer, politician—will only make your health worse.

So stop resisting and start moving.

Everyone, even those who are obese or disabled, can move more. All it takes is making the decision to do so. Even if you feel your schedule is crammed to the limit, you still can add much needed physical activity to your daily routine without overloading your schedule further or breaking the back of your day. If you are used to rising from bed, rushing to get dressed, grabbing a cup of coffee, and rushing out the door, stop, and look at your morning again.

- Greet the day with a stretch and a smile: (If you can't manage the smile, at least manage to stretch.) Try getting up 5 minutes earlier and doing a series of stretching exercises. For example, lying in bed, stretch one arm overhead, arching your back and stretching your legs at the same time. Then do the same with the other arm. And remember that smiling uses less than half the facial muscles that frowning requires. Smiling, then, is actually easier.

Warming up and Cooling Down

We've all heard this good advice plenty of times, and yet few of us heed it—even as we age and our bones and joints start calling out, with greater frequency, "Hey, take it easy," and those aches and pains come sooner and last longer. So, let me tell you, once more with feeling: Warming up before you exercise and cooling down afterward are indispensable to ensuring the safety of any exercise routine. They are required, not optional, elements of your workout.

If you are just a "no-good-nick" when it comes to warming up and cooling down and consider these gentle moments of your workout a waste of time, you might try taking an exercise class with an instructor or using a quality exercise video at home. Exercise instructors and physical trainers always include a warm-up and cool-down part of every class, because they know how important these stretches are to avoiding injury.

Warming Up

Stretching exercises that are done slowly protect against injury to your muscles, ligaments, and tendons. The experts vary on how long you should spend warming up, but at least a 10 minute warm-up is recommended. But, hey, if you can only stand 5 minutes, in this case, it's better than nothing. The goal of the warm-up stretches is to maximize muscle flexibility. Warm, flexible muscles are much less likely to sustain injury. A "warm" muscle is one in which the blood flow has been increased from its resting position. When warming up, your pulse will also rise, as will your body temperature. Never bounce or jerk your body during your warm-up. You'll do more harm

- Walk, don't ride: We all think we're saving time when we drive, take a taxi, or take the bus, but we may be losing time in the long run. The more you use your body, the better your health, and the greater your chances of longevity. Think always of when you might be able to park your car further away from your destination; better yet, leave your car at home and walk to where you need to go. Ten blocks or half a mile is better than nothing, and a mile or more is the beginning of a good day's investment in taking care of yourself.
- Keep barbells at your desk: Keep a set of free weights at your desk at work. Use whatever weights are comfortable

than good. Your warm-up should concentrate on the muscle you'll be using most during your workout, but you should stretch all major muscle groups. Warm up gradually to avoid over stretching your muscles—that's why your warm-up should be longer, not shorter.

Cooling Down

Cooling down is equally important as warming up. Once again experts vary on the amount of time you should devote to cooling down, but 10 minutes is a good, average recommendation. And once again, any time is better than none. Never walk away from an exercise routine without doing some stretching. That's like cold turkey—too hard, in this case, on your muscles. Cooling down prevents cramping, as well as preventing injury. Interestingly,

cooling down also increases the blood flow to your heart—a good thing, as Martha Stewart would say, since your heart has been pumping out all that good blood to help you pump those muscles.

To cool down, start by decreasing your pace gradually in whatever exercise you are doing. If you've been jogging, this means slowing to a walk. If you've been bicycling, this means not taking any hills, but peddling easily on flat ground. You should never stop exercising suddenly. Once you've gradually halted your aerobic activity, then begin your cool-down stretches. You can use the same stretches you used warming up, making sure you pay attention to each major muscle group. Massaging your muscles for a moment or two can also help to prevent cramping.

for you, even 2 or 3 pounders are better than none. When you're on the phone, alternate doing bicep curls with your left and right arms. You can do this either sitting at your desk, as long as you can extend each arm completely to begin the exercise, or standing. If you're on a long, boring phone call, you may even get in two or three sets of ten repetitions apiece.

- Engage in phone-ercise: Personally, I think cell phones are highly overrated and would dearly love to start a restaurant solely to put at the bottom of the menu, "Pipes and cigars welcome. Cell phones not welcome." But modern technology aside, few of us are bound by cord and plug to our telephones these days. Therefore, you get another opportunity to stay in motion and one less excuse not to do so. When the phone rings, stand up, answer it, and start moving.

- Engage in dirty dancing or housework to a beat: Even housework—unsexy, unattractive housework—does

Finding Your Target Heart Rate

The whole point of aerobic exercise is to make your heart beat faster, thereby improving your cardiovascular fitness. A person who is out of condition basically is forcing his or her heart to beat more frequently than the person who is well conditioned. Over a 24-hour period, the sedentary person's heart might beat as much as forty thousand times more than the conditioned person's heart—think of it, forty thousand times. That's a lot more work for your heart. One of the first results of getting in shape is to lower your heart rate, thus giving your heart a rest.

To make this happen, you must calculate your target heart rate zone (THRZ). Then, when exercising, you must hold to a pace that keeps your heart in that zone long enough to reap the benefits of aerobic exercise.

The experts vary on recommending an ideal THRZ, but that's not unusual. Experts vary on everything. In general, most experts agree that approximately 70 percent of your maximal heart rate is a reasonable target zone.

Calculating your target heart rate is fairly simple. First, subtract your age from 220. (Men in unbe-

burn calories. I like to put on my Walkman and add a little extra motion to the whole affair by dancing through the bathroom, the kitchen, the vacuuming, and the bed making. It's an almost entertaining way to get a necessary job done and get some exercise.

THE WHOLE 9 YARDS

Just when you thought it was safe to go back in the comfortable water of your sedentary life, that shark fin in constant motion is telling you that getting moving is not enough. Getting moving is better than nothing, but once you've done this, you'll need to challenge yourself again, if you really want to become and stay healthy.

A complete exercise program depends on combining anaerobic and aerobic exercise with exercises that enhance flexibility and balance. Now that you've gotten yourself moving and have gotten a little rush of adrenaline and pride by meeting this first

lievable condition—who probably don't have diabetes—should subtract from 205.) Then calculate 70 percent of that number. If you are 40 years old, your THRZ would be 70 percent of 180, or 126. If you've led a sedentary life for a long time and already have some complications related to diabetes, even minor ones, your doctor will want you to work with a much lower target heart rate as you begin, probably 50 percent or even less, depending on your individual situation. Your job is to maintain your target heart rate during the intensive portion of your exercise routing.

Taking Your Pulse

You should take your pulse, before, during, and after your routine, to ensure your reach your target heart rate and to ensure that your heart rate decreases appropriately after your cool down. Taking your pulse is easy. All you do is press your index and middle fingers on your wrist, close to the thumb joint. Then count the number of beats for 15 seconds and multiply by four to find a 1-minute reading.

goal, it's time to tell you you've only just begun. Don't get depressed; it will get easier as you go along.

STARTING SAFELY

No diabetic should begin an exercise regimen, no matter how conservative, without the hearty approval of his or her doctor. Even if you were not diabetic, your doctor would tell you to begin slowly, but surely. Most diabetics can increase their level of physical activity, as long as they proceed sensibly, with their doctor's okay and guidance.

Every diabetic should have a physical checkup before beginning an exercise program. Your doctor will give you a complete physical evaluation, which will include checking your blood pressure, your circulation, and your cholesterol level. If you have had diabetes for some time, your doctor will also want to check your eyes and your feet. Long-term diabetics sometimes suffer from retinopathy, an eye condition that involves the presence of very fragile blood vessels in the eye. Long-term diabetics may also suffer from neuropathy and have foot problems exacerbated by the neuropathy, such as infections or foot ulcers. The doctor will also check your family history to see if you are at risk for heart disease or any other conditions in addition to diabetes. If you are overweight or obese, your doctor will probably recommend a very gradual but consistent introduction of physical activity into your life.

Your doctor's recommendations will depend on how long you have been a diabetic, whether or not you have maintained good control of blood sugar levels, and whether or not you have developed any complications. Whether you are overweight will also influence your doctor's recommendations. One reminder— if you are a diabetic, your warm-up and cool-down periods are essential to avoiding problems. To protect your heart and prevent injury, never start exercising without warming up and never, never stop exercising without cooling down after your workout. Your heart has been working overtime, pumping all that extra blood to oxygenate your muscles. Give your heart a chance to recuperate and get its "blood bearings" back. This is a bit of a stretch, but stretching is good—you would probably do better simply warming up and cooling down than you would exercising full tilt without a warm-up and cool-down period.

When to Stop Exercising

If you notice any of the following symptoms during your workout, you should stop immediately:

- Heart palpitations
- Dizziness or faintness

- Shortness of breath
- Blurred vision
- Foot pain
- Pain running down your left arm
- Neck pain
- Nausea

Except in extreme cases, the unavoidable truth is that it is usually not exercise that will hurt you but the lack of exercise that is slowly but surely destroying your health. Work with your doctor to find a safe exercise plan, and your health and self-image are bound to improve.

When you do begin an exercise routine, track your blood glucose levels very carefully. If they begin to become elevated or consistently lower, consult your doctor. This may simply be a period of adjustment, or you may need to regulate your diet when you exercise or change your routine (see If You Are Taking Insulin or OHAs). Also drink plenty of water to avoid dehydration, which can also affect blood sugar. If you have even very slight neuropathy, pay particular attention to the care of your feet and examine them after every workout.

IF YOU ARE TAKING INSULIN OR OHAs

If you do take medication, stabilizing blood sugar before you begin to work out should be an important part of your routine.

To do this, you'll have to rely on carbohydrates for help. This is the one exception to the rule of minimizing carbohydrate intake. To find the right amount of carbohydrate to "protect" your blood glucose levels and avoid hypoglycemia (low blood sugar), you'll need to use your blood testing kit religiously and experiment. If you are of average weight, the rule of thumb is that your blood sugar will rise approximately 5 mg/dL per gram of carbohydrate.

Many Type I diabetics use fruits or sweets to keep blood glucose levels from falling dramatically. In fact, until recently, this was standard practice in the treatment of diabetes. According to Dr. Richard K. Bernstein, however, the end result after the exercise is usually a rise in blood glucose levels. He recommends, instead, taking glucose tablets, and his choice as the most efficient glucose tablets is Dextrotabs. They work quickly, beginning to raise blood sugar in 3 minutes and ending after about 40 minutes—just right for a workout. They are available through most pharmacies and from diabetes mail-order companies.

ALL I NEED NOW IS A SPRAINED ANKLE: HOW TO AVOID INJURY

The most common injuries while exercising are due to excessive demands placed on muscles and/or other tissues and bones, and they are caused most frequently by not warming up and cooling down properly. Minimizing your risk of injury involves, first of all, setting realistic goals for yourself. If you were a championship ice skater 20 years ago, don't go out on the ice for the first time planning to land a double axle, or a single axle, for that matter. By the same token, if you're an ex-basketball jock, don't go for the perfect slam dunk in the first minute of play. You're likely to pull a hamstring you may have almost forgotten you had.

When you begin to add exercise to your life, start slow, and build up your routine gradually. If you plan to become a regular jogger but haven't been running for a while, start with two or three 20- to 30-minute workouts per week and alternate between jogging and walking for 10- or 5-minute intervals (if 10 minutes of jogging is too strenuous). Should you become short of breath or notice any pain or strain, you should stop immediately. Within 2 weeks, you should be up to jogging 30 minutes without stopping and, with any luck, be injury free.

Here are some commonsense rules that will help you avoid injury:

- Always consult your doctor before beginning an exercise routine. If you have been exercising and are planning to changes sports or disciplines, you should also consult your doctor.
- Keep track of blood glucose levels every time you work out. If any significant changes occur, call your doctor.
- If you already suffer from one or more diabetic complications work out your exercise plan with the supervision of your doctor, paying particular attention to foot gear and the stress and strain of exercise on your feet. If any problems arise, contact him or her immediately. Even a minor complaint could have major consequences, if you don't attend to it.
- If you are new to a sport or discipline, seek instruction from a professional trainer or sports instructor. Even one lesson will help reduce your risk of injury. If you feel you can't afford the investment, at least read up on your chosen activity before beginning.
- Always warm up and cool down. This is extremely important for diabetics (see Warming up and Cooling Down).

- Don't strain. When you work out, you should feel that you are working, but not working too hard.
- Choose the proper shoe for your sport or activity—one that will protect you against injury.
- Make sure you exercise on a surface with some amount of "give." A hard surface increases the stress on muscles and bones and raises the risk of injury. Grass or dirt are better than concrete for running (as long as you are running on level ground). A wood floor or a padded floor is better for aerobic dancing than concrete or industrial carpeting (which may cause you to stumble).
- Learn proper form. Make sure you are trained in how to properly perform the exercise you choose. Good form helps prevent injury and helps you get the greatest benefit from your workout.
- Remember to pace yourself. Know your limits and never overexert yourself.
- Be aware of your body. If you feel extremely fatigued, stop.
- Breathe deeply and regularly. Believe it or not, many of us tend to hold our breath when concentrating intensely on our exercise routine. This is not good. So be aware of your breathing and consciously remind yourself to breathe in deeply through the nose and exhale through the mouth.
- Work out regularly and frequently. Those who exercise sporadically are far more likely to condemn themselves to injury.
- Increase the pace and duration of your routine gradually. In other words, be patient with yourself. Don't expect to

be running 5 miles by the end of week one, and don't expect to be running a 4-minute mile by the end of the week either.

- The longer the duration of your workout, the better. Because you are a diabetic, short intervals of aerobic exercise can raise your blood sugar. Thus, running for 10 minutes is far less beneficial to your overall health than jogging for 30 to 40 minutes. If your busy schedule makes you feel cramped for time, better to work out 3 days a week for 45 minutes to an hour, than 5 days a week for 20 minutes. On your "off" days, make walking at a brisk pace for 40 minutes a goal for the day.
- Don't compete. March to the beat of your own drummer. The race is not to the swift, in this case, but to the steady. And, anyway, there is no race. When we try to outdo, we all have a tendency to overdo. Remember, you're not going for a medal; you're going for the gold in health. Playing it safe is part of ensuring good health when exercising.
- If you do suffer an injury, take care of it right away. Particularly because you are a diabetic, you don't want to neglect an injury and run the risk of further complicating your medical care. Attend to strains and sprains immediately to avoid a chronic condition. Attend to cuts immediately to avoid infection.
- Never exercise in extreme heat or cold or at an altitude you are not used to.
- Touch base with your doctor periodically. Remember, even if you are symptom-free and complication-free, you're still a diabetic. Be cautious, not cavalier.

"Spinning"

The first time I heard about spinning, I thought it was some sort of weird folk dancing inspired by the dervishes in Turkey and done by women who otherwise would be dancing with wolves—or something like that. But it's nothing of the kind.

Spinning is a new high-tech way to use stationary bicycles. And spinning is one of the most intensive aerobic workouts you can get in 45 minutes. And most importantly, you use the bike at a high-resistance level for most of the workout. Your instructor will call this part "climbing the hill," which is probably what appeals to me, loving Sisyphus as I do. As you make your arduous climb, you will be burning glucose while getting a tremendous aerobic workout—a perfect balance for the diabetic.

Most gyms now offer spinning classes with loud music to keep you entertained and occupied while you test your endurance. The music keeps you from getting bored and makes the class go faster. Also, once you get your sneakers strapped into your toe clips, your far less likely to go to all the trouble it will take you to quit early. Take it slow in the beginning; you'll find your stamina building after just 2 weeks of two classes per week. My blood sugar afterward is about 115–120 mg/dL—the best it's been after any aerobic workout. (One tip: Always use a little more resistance, not less, to keep burning that glucose.)

THE NON IDENTICAL TWINS OF GOOD HEALTH: ANAEROBIC AND AEROBIC EXERCISE

Now that you're moving, and not sitting still, and walking, if not running, it's time to complicate your life once again and give you another challenge. Just when you thought it was safe to manage a weekly aerobic activity schedule for cardiovascular fitness, now there's another shark in the water—anaerobic exercise. Anaerobic exercise is necessary to build muscle strength and ever so important for the diabetic, because it burns eighteen times the glucose that aerobic exercise burns—yes, eighteen times. And I am not a snake oil salesman.

Aerobic exercise strengthens the heart, helps maintain a healthy immune system, and increases endurance—all good. It can, however, raise blood glucose levels if you exert yourself strenuously for only a short time. The point is not to give up aerobic exercise but to tailor it to your needs as a diabetic (exercising over a longer period of time at a lower level of exertion), and to add anaerobic exercise to your life.

Anaerobic means without oxygen, which means the activity you are engaging in does not necessitate substantial addition of oxygen and, therefore, does not raise your heart rate significantly. Hence, as beneficial as anaerobic exercise and activity is to your health, it will not take the place of aerobic exercise; we all know the motto of good health: Raise your heart rate regularly but don't raise your blood pressure. What anaerobic exercise can do, however, is to strengthen your muscles and increase the amount of muscle mass, which, alas, we lose naturally as we grow older.

Anaerobic exercise may also be referred to as static activity and depends on increasing resistance. Chopping wood or carrying heavy boxes are examples of anaerobic activity. However, if you don't do manual labor for a living and you don't heat your house with firewood, there are other means of accruing the strengthening and conditioning benefits of anaerobic exercise. These include free weights, rubber exercise bands that increase resistance during exercise routines, and weight machines.

I find the way to ensure that I get regular anaerobic exercise is to keep a set of free weights at home. I've worked up to 6-pound barbells, which I use for a 10- to 15-minute routine about five times a week. I follow a video called "Crunch" (produced by a local gym in New York City) and have even come to depend on the monotonous but perky trainer instructing me on what to do next. I think of her as my "poor woman's personal trainer." We have one TV, and it's in my son's room. After I take him to school in the morning, I do my routine right away, to avoid finding rationalization for not doing it. Then I catch a little Sesame Street on my son's TV before getting down to work. Five minutes of Sesame Street can be great for your mental health.

Now that I've pretty much memorized the routine, I'll do my sets and repetitions when I'm wandering around talking on my portable phone or taking a break from writing or listening to the news on National Public Radio. You'll find that once you get the hang of a few exercises for upper and lower body strength, you can incorporate them into your day, without having to rearrange your life much at all.

If you have the money to belong to a health club, all the better. You can use the weight machines there. I recommend shelling out the money for one or two training sessions with a coach or trainer or whatever the instructors in your gym of choice are called. A qualified instructor can help you establish a routine that is appropriate for your level of expertise.

A Meditation on Walking

Even though walking is the activity that gets us around and we really couldn't do without it, we really don't give walking enough credit. Walking is good for the body and good for the soul. Walking is practical—it gets us from here to there—and walking is free. Walking even takes its place in the canon of world philosophy. To paraphrase the declaration of one of the world's great philosophers, Kierkegaard, "Every walk is a good walk."

Every walk is a good walk is about as true as the truth gets. However, this does not mean that every walk you take can count as your quota of exercise for the day. For that you need to walk and then some. For walking to qualify as aerobic activity, you need to walk briskly without stopping. Thus, the start and stop walking we do when doing errands doesn't count in the scheme of aerobic activity. In addition, if walking is your exercise of choice, you'll have to walk for longer periods of time than you would jog or run or bicycle, because it takes more time to raise your heart rate to your target heart rate zone when walking.

These are hardly caveats, though. Walking is still one of the finest, most useful activities there is. It is a particularly useful way to re-enter the world of the moving, if you have been sedentary for a long time. It is also a good choice

AN ANAEROBIC "LOW" IS A DIABETIC'S "HIGH"

Just as nothing can replace aerobic activity when it comes to the benefits accrued by the cardiovascular system, so nothing can equal anaerobic activity when it comes to aiding your body in keeping blood glucose levels stabilized. As mentioned previously, anaerobic exercise burns eighteen times the glucose that aerobic activity does. Thus, by incorporating an anaerobic exercise routine into your life, you can actually lower blood glucose levels over time.

The Glucose Is in the "Burn"

Remember, the more you feel the resistance ("the burn"), the greater the anaerobic benefit and, therefore, the greater the amount of glucose you're using. The greater the weights you use, the greater the resistance, and the more glucose you burn.

of activity if you are overweight or obese. The risk of injury and accident is low, and you can almost always get an okay from your doctor to walk, even if you have a heart condition.

Walking is particularly good for diabetics, especially long walks, as it raises the heart rate slowly and does not cause an immediate rise in blood glucose levels. More strenuous exercise, such as running or tennis, done for only a brief period of time, can actually raise blood glucose levels. This occurs because strenuous exercise causes the release of certain counter-regulatory or "stress" hormones, which can trigger the liver to convert glycogen into glucose, sending more glucose into the bloodstream. So, the longer you walk or perform any strenuous exercise, the better your chances for normal blood glucose levels during exercise.

For those of us Type A personalities who find that our stress level rises when we try to relax, walking can also be relaxing and a great stress reliever. If, however, you are afraid that much time with yourself might be frightening or if you find walking boring, try walking with a friend or investing in a Walkman and some music or a book on tape that you've been meaning to read. When it comes to walking, there is no excuse not to do it. So, what are you waiting for? Get up and walk.

The same goes for repetitions and sets—the more you do, the more you burn.

A Little Weight Can Mean a Lot

When it comes to weight lifting, anyone can do it. If you're thinking you would have to be bench pressing a hefty load to reap the anaerobic benefits, think again.

You can use one of two types of weights in your weight training program, either free weights or machines. There are two types of free weights—dumbbells, which are held in one hand, and barbells, which require a two-handed grip. Dumbbells and barbells are easy to use, easy to store, and inexpensive to purchase. Before you invest in a set of dumbbells or barbells, however, you should consult a qualified trainer regarding what the appropriate weight is for your size and strength. To aid in gripping your weights, you may also want to buy a pair of training gloves. But don't bother investing in one of those training belts you see the macho folk, male and female, parading around in at the gym. Recent studies have shown that these belts provide no extra support. They're merely cosmetic accessories in which to make the gym social scene.

Most gyms feature a myriad of weight-training machines for you to choose from. You can also purchase weight-training machines to use at home. And as weight training increases in popularity, more and more inexpensive models of these machines are becoming available.

What Is a Repetition? What Is a Set?

The structure of an anaerobic weight-training routine includes repetitions and sets. A repetition, or "rep," refers to the execution of one complete "lift." (A lift refers to any weight-lifting movement.) A "set" is a series of "reps" done without stopping between any of the "reps." For a workout to be productive, you should strive to accomplish at least three sets comprised of between eight to twelve repetitions. Remember, too, that we diabetics want to maximize resistance, because this is how you burn the most glucose. This means increasing the amount of weight you are using as soon as you are comfortable doing so and maximizing your workout by doing more "sets" as soon as you are able to. The more resistance and the more reps, the more glucose you burn.

ACCENTUATE THE NEGATIVE

In any "rep," the "negative" part of any motion refers to the half of the exercise in which you are returning the weight to its original position. It is during the "negative" part of the motion that most injuries occur, when greater stress is put on the tendons. So you want to pay attention to this part of your routine. Remember to let the weight down at the same rate that you lifted it. This will protect you from injury, and it will also help you get the maximum benefit. Rushing through the negative portion of the repetition will only rob your muscles of this benefit.

CREATING YOUR OWN CUSTOMIZED EXERCISE REGIMEN

As with all areas of self-improvement, once again, it's not going to work if you set impossible challenges and goals for yourself or if you fool yourself into believing for a day or two that you really will stick to an exercise routine you hate. If you go with the old cliché "Pay your dues," you are far more likely to pay for a day and then quit than if you stick with the new mantra "Invest in yourself." Investing means that any little bit counts, and, eventually, those little bits do add up.

CROSS-TRAINING

Simply put, cross-training means not doing the same thing for aerobic exercise all the time. So alternate. Don't do the same thing all the time. The best way to fight injury (and boredom) is to avoid doing the same exercise routine over and over. It's that simple, even if it sounds hip.

AEROBIC OPTIONS

These days there are almost as many forms of exercise to choose from as there are Web sites on the Internet. Well, not

Yoga for Body, Blood Sugar, Heart, and Mind

Though the recent, trendy popularity of yoga may make those of us who scorn fads and shun the cream of popular culture a little suspicious, I have to say that in this case, the popularity and praise the discipline of yoga is now enjoying is well deserved.

The benefits of yoga cannot be over-rated. It is good for the body, the mind, and the soul. Even practicing a series of yoga postures as infrequently as twice a week will help you increase your flexibility and lower your stress level. Yoga can also be beneficial in improving your sense of balance and in helping you to breathe more deeply—another factor in relieving stress.

While you practice the postures, you will be working your muscles, developing good balance, and increasing flexibility, and you will also find that the tension you brought to class will begin to diminish. When you inhale and exhale is essential to the performance of each posture, so you will find that you are naturally breathing more deeply as you perform the postures. The instructor will also help you to focus on calming your thoughts and turning down the noise level in your head as you move from posture to posture. Yoga is also particularly helpful in strengthening and protecting the back, and because of the concentration on breathing, it can also be very helpful if you suffer from asthma.

The postures are called asanas. Although they stretch and strengthen the body, they are not calisthenics; they are components of the overall spiritual discipline that is yoga. In addition to being beneficial to your overall physical and mental health, yoga is also an interesting discipline to study, and the poses have quite wonderful names. In one 20-minute session, you may find yourself turning from a fish into a cobra. The postures fall into essentially two categories: forward bending poses and backward bending poses. There are

quite. But in any case, you can choose from a vast array of aerobic options from walking or jogging or bicycle riding to in-line skating or aerobic dance classes or boxing. And you can vary your routine according to the seasons, choosing ice skating, skiing, or cross-country skiing in the winter, if you live in the country, and running or swimming in the summer.

ANAEROBIC OPTIONS

You should manage three to four anaerobic workouts per week. Whether these are done at home to a videotape or

also poses that focus specifically on breathing. The poses form a sort of yin and yang of positions that build flexibility, and moving from the backward-bending to the forward-bending postures helps to protect against injury.

You can find a comprehensive guide to yoga postures in any bookstore, and there are also a number of videos available by trained yoga instructors. In addition, many gyms and fitness centers offer classes in yoga. I tend to prefer the classes offered by traditional yoga centers because they focus more on the spiritual and calming effects of the discipline. Yoga is not supposed to be competitive, and the classes offered in fitness centers often end up being more achievement oriented than not. While they may offer sensible instruction on the postures, they focus a little too much on "pumping muscles" and are a bit lacking on the concepts of discipline, peace, and tranquillity. But, each to his own sun salutation.

One interesting note: The shoulder stand, called "the queen of the poses," is said to have many benefits. It is considered beneficial to your thyroid and your pancreas, as those organs are massaged while you rise into the position and remain there. Whether or not this is valid would be hard to prove, but the notion makes me love the shoulder stand a little more than I already do. In any case, "the queen of the poses" is definitely good for your circulation, and improving circulation is important for all diabetics. As long as you do not suffer from a neck or back problem or eye problems, you may find the shoulder stand both restful and stimulating.

Finally, where else can you transform from cow to cat to downward dog to cobra, fish, and crow and back to yourself in an hour? Traveling through such identities can be spiritually lifting and refreshing in the midst of a busy day.

improvised from an anaerobic workout manual or the exercises offered here (see Free Weights Any Time of Day) doesn't matter, as long as you do it. Or you can go to a gym and use the weight machines there, if you cannot motivate yourself at home.

Also remember to add anaerobic activity to your life in general—carry the groceries home yourself, shovel the snow, chop the wood, carry the laundry upstairs. All of these are resistance activities.

YOUR WEEKLY SCHEDULE

Once again, always remember to warm up before and cool down after any exercise routine. Try to vary what you do for exercise and try to do some form of exercise every day. Cross-training can help. A sample plan might go as follows:

- Running or bicycling: Run or ride a bike two times a week, 40 minutes per session—either outdoors or on a stationary bicycle. (If you run, use swimming as your cross-training exercise to help prevent injury to your joints.)
- Swimming or aerobic dance: Swim or dance one to two times a week. Remember, though, that if you have foot ulcers or any other complications regarding your feet, the water can cause maceration of the skin, and, therefore, swimming is not a choice for you. (If you swim, use aerobic dance as your cross-training exercise, since weight-resistant exercise helps prevent osteoporosis.)
- Weights: Lift weights two to three times a week, 20 to 30 minutes per workout. If you can't do this, at least use your free weights around the house or at your desk.

If all of this sounds like too much, try the following:

- Speed walking: Build up to walking about 40 minutes, three times a week, using light free weights as you do so to increase your resistance activity.
- Free weights: Use a beginner's free weight video three times a week and try to complete the video using light weights to begin and building up to heavier weights as you become adept at your routine.

Calories Burned for Various Sports and Activities

Activity	Calories/Hour	Impact
Aerobic Dance	350	Low
Basketball	560	High
Cycling	315	L
Gardening	350	L/H
Jogging/6mph	700	H
Raking Leaves	280	L
Softball	350	L/H
Skiing (cross country)	490	L
Skiing (downhill)	350	L/H
Swimming (most strokes)	420	L
Tai chi	280	L
Tennis	490	H
Walking (moderate pace)	250	L
Weight training	420	L
Yoga	280	L

MOTIVATION FOR THE NEW MILLENNIUM

To make any life change stick, your resolve has to last for a lifetime. This means through other unexpected, even unwanted, life changes, through all the changes in your path you did not plan on and all the curves life is bound to toss your way. The aim is not only normal blood sugar now; it's normal blood sugar next year and into the next century.

We are all only as good as our motivation. So goes our motivation, so go we. This means how "good" we are varies daily. I don't know anyone who is 100 percent motivated 365 days of the year. And if there is such a person, I don't want to know him or her.

So staying motivated is key. If you don't believe me, then, as Jack Paar would say, "We've got nothing." And staying motivated means striking a balance between when we give into our sloth-like selves and our driven selves. If you drive yourself until you can't stand it anymore, you're likely to rebel by indulging in too much time off—"I deserve it" being the operative credo. On the other hand, if you always take time off and indulge, you'll never get started. A little self-indulgence is the handmaiden of staying happily motivated, but a lot is motivation's destroyer.

To ensure you stay motivated, begin your new regime slowly. A "New You" has never been built in a day. And if your expectations don't jive with your present condition and skill level, you're sure to be back in the Barcalounger before you can say "warm-up exercises." Remember, when it comes to adding exercise to your life, gradual changes have a far greater chance of sticking than sudden bursts of manic overhauling. So start slow and keep going.

Make sure before you begin that you've made exercise choices that you can feel enthusiastic about, maybe even enjoy. If you like to walk, walk. If you like to walk but get bored, use a Walkman and listen to music or books on tape. If you love to row but don't live by the Thames or any other great river, buy a rowing machine.

The following may help you stick to it for the long term:

- Exercise with a friend. The buddy system has been proven to be one of the most efficient ways to get more people off their behinds and into exercise. If you choose a buddy who is less motivated than you are, choose a second friend and alternate. Don't let a lazy friend infect you with the same disease.
- Don't allow yourself any excuses. Exercise is part of your life, now, not simply an option to choose or reject.
- Set reasonable goals.
- Remember that change is good and that boredom is bad. If you get bored with your routine, change activities. Recently I discovered "spinning"—high-speed stationary biking. The instructor was inspiring. The music was exciting. The workout was terrific. My motivation returned, and for now I'm addicted. When this wanes, I'm sure I'll find some other form of exercise to keep me motivated to work out.
- Momentum helps. Once you set an exercise schedule, stick to it. Try not to skip exercising when you've planned to, unless you're sick. Getting into the habit is like hitting your stride—the getting there gets easier.
- Think of your exercise plan the way you do your investment planning or your retirement plan. You're investing in the future. Over time, even when investing in small increments, the benefits to your "health account" will accrue.
- Treat yourself—not to a sugar-coated donut but to an evening out with friends, a movie, a long-distance chat with an old friend, that new software or CD you've been wanting, or some new exercise gear.

part 6

Methodology Over Matter: Contributions to a Centered Life

If you have been working on your own customized program for managing your diabetes while you have been reading this book, there are two possible results. Either you're making some very positive progress in improving your health or you're in abject despair and disillusioned by the whole prospect of trying to make a difference in your own life. We're going to disregard the latter possibility, because it's too depressing, and focus on the former, which is the kind of uplifting result we're aiming for here. And it is uplifting. Hard as the heavy lifting might have been, there is nothing quite like the sense of peaceful power you get from making a positive change in your own life. From my own experience, I can say that while it might not be as rapturous as all that, it is exhilarating. You may not have won the Olympics or a Nobel prize, but you have done something inarguably significant—you've altered a biological fact, used your mind, your determination, your self-discipline, and all that other good stuff to engineer a profound effect on your body. Matter may not be created or destroyed, but matter can be altered. From high blood glucose to lower blood glucose levels, you've managed a feat that only decades ago was seen as impossible. Congratulations!

You'll find that your accomplishment will begin to subtly influence other aspects of your life and that your personal refrain is "Well if I can do that, I truly can do anything." And remember, you're not different because you're a diabetic, you're healthier.

15

Maintenance Is Everything

From people to space stations, gardens to automobiles, it's always maintenance. We humans hate this hard and unforgiving truth because as much as we want to keep going, we don't want to do the boring, humdrum, time-consuming work it takes to keep going well.

Now you have to. But as time goes on, you'll see that it gets easier, because feeling good becomes its own motivation.

TIGHT CONTROL IN AN OUT-OF-CONTROL WORLD

Not long into my new way of life, it occurred to me that managing my diabetes had a restorative effect on my beleaguered peace of mind. The froth of daily events still besieged my powers of concentration, and the shrapnel of life's challenges scattered itself all over my positive attitude, but like a boat with a solid mooring, I didn't drift too far. My Glucometer was my medical confessional. After the agitation of any given crisis, there was my blood to check. This meant that no rationalizations I might create could pass muster with the lancet and the test strip. If I ate only a handful of macadamia nuts one evening, the evidence would be there 2 hours postprandial—a ten to twenty point rise in my bgl. This also meant, however, that having confessed, I could start again, if not exactly fresh. This continuum of personal honesty had a steadying effect on my life that was as comforting as it was stabilizing and helped to make personal maintenance not only possible but also a permanent part of my life. My goals—normal blood sugar and a small amplitude—keep me company.

Playing the Course

We all need our mythologies to get through. And let's face it, a little romanticizing can go a long way in turning what could be only daily drudgery into a noble quest. With a little finessing, a few apposite images, the horizon can expand and conforming to a restrictive diet can become a transformative experience. And any time restrictions can be converted into the path toward inner discipline, you are going to be more likely to stay the course and not rebel. Rebellion directly undercuts long-term tight control of diabetes. And whatever helps get you through the night with levels of 110 or under, mythologies, mantras, and metaphors should be seen as equally important as anaerobic exercise or a healthy low-carbohydrate meal.

For me, the game and the metaphor is golf, and the day is my course. Though I'm actually a baseball fan, golf works better for this analogy. Golf is a game that demands patience and at which a player can only excel over time. It is a game of details and nuances, chess on a green board. While the single shot can be paramount, the overall game is key. No one shot does you in. No one shot saves you. A good chip shot, a great putt, even a hole in one are worth little in the scheme of things if they are not unified by a winning strategy that includes personal humility after sinking the 20-foot putt, determination after winding up in a sand trap, the practiced skill to make a comeback, and the perseverance to endure the ups and downs inherent in any round of golf. Golf is a game in which big mistakes demand major corrections and minor mistakes take a much lesser toll—a steady unspectacular game brings you into the clubhouse with a lower score than an erratic game that contains bursts of excellence. Finally, in golf, you play the course, and, ultimately, you play yourself, again and again, over and over—much like diabetes and much like life.

WHY THOMAS JEFFERSON WOULD HAVE BEEN A MODEL DIABETIC

We all know that the great Thomas Jefferson knew lots about a great number of subjects, but he knew even more than we know he knew. This was a man who was a radical thinker for his time or any time and who was equally unconventional in his personal health remedies (soaking your feet in ice water every day?); he was, in the overall, as balanced as they come. Exercise, food, wine, the company of friends, creativity of spirit were always a part of his life. So was balance. So was moderation. So was discipline. He made all three a part of his life. And he understood, profoundly, the necessity to redefine restriction as self-discipline and made self-discipline a permanent personal quest.

In addition, the physical world was as important to him as the world of the mind. He ate a diet rich in protein, and of course, he didn't have to worry about additives and preservatives. The carbohydrates of which he partook were largely vegetables grown on his farm and whole grains. He imbibed fine wines in a more moderate manner than many of his contemporaries. (I believe he sipped some sherry and some port now and again, off limits for us.) He touted the benefits of exercise and was a living example of what he preached, embracing a life filled with physical activities. He did love those peas he grew in his garden—not on our list—but in general he lived a perfect example of prevention in action.

As you can see from my choice of epigraph, I admire the guy, and with good reason. First and foremost, he knew that "Eternal vigilance is the price of liberty." You're much better off after you realize that even freedom doesn't come free. This works equally well when considering the freedom of intellectual thought or the physical freedom good health allows. *Vigilance* must be the watchword for every diabetic who is managing tight control.

In addition, Thomas Jefferson never valued the life of the mind over the life of the body. If one hand washes the other, then body and mind depend on each other, and this great statesman knew it was important to cultivate both. True, he was something of a gentlemen of leisure with the exceptional grounds and charm of Monticello making daily life a tad more idyllic and easy on the soul. But remember that he designed the masterpiece himself and was always involved in every aspect of the building and maintenance of his now historic home. And though a gentleman of leisure, he was never sedentary. Your body can do at least something with what you eat even if your diet isn't as healthy as it should be, but muscle, bone, and joint can do nothing with a static state. If you are sedentary, the only active thing you are doing is contributing to the deterioration of every muscle (including your heart), bone, and joint in your body.

In most realms of life (other than the sexual), Jefferson was a man who paid attention to detail, which every diabetic must do in order to stick to his or her regimen. Normal blood glucose levels are in the details.

And Thomas Jefferson, though not a diabetic, took care of his feet. He understood that above all else, our feet get us there (wherever *there* is). Despite the ice water at 6 A.M. (or whatever ungodly hour it was), he had the right idea. He took his boots off. He bathed and cared for his feet, unlike most of his contemporaries. Imagine those eighteenth-century feet, many of them in boots for 24 hours or more at a stretch? I'd rather not.

President Jefferson also had a gourmet's palate and a love of food, but he was a gourmet, not a glutton. (We hope this is true in his taste in women, too). He appreciated tastes and unusual recipes, but he did not abuse his palate by overindulging. (There are those peas, which we wouldn't eat, but it's a small transgression.) Clearly, Thomas Jefferson had other areas in life in which he partook more than many thought he should have, but who are we to judge? Those of us who must face our blood sugar failures as well as the rest of our, well . . . shortcomings? I'm not one.

As aforesaid, he also liked his wine . . . but not to excess. He enjoyed it as a delicious accompaniment to a fine meal, something to graciously offer friends, a digestive, and a social pleasure—once again, a perfect balance.

And as one of the framers of the Declaration of Independence and the Constitution of the United States, he shaped and crafted documents whose power has endured for more than two centuries. Talk about maintenance. And about his taste in women—I recommend him whether his memory cures or not.

Above all, he participated in life, which we can do to the fullest when we are in our best shape. Life, liberty, and the pursuit of happiness will be more assuredly yours when you take control of your diabetes.

A Quasi-Parable on Faith, Thomas Jefferson, Lewis and Clark, and Diabetes

President Jefferson was a great buff of Western legend and lore, and his impressive library held almost everything ever written on the West at the time. In fact, he had a greater collection of Western lore than anyone on this earth. It must be remembered that way back then, the United States of America was strictly an eastern seaboard proposition, and everything beyond those thirteen states was fairly much a vast, unexplored territory called the wilderness or just the West. And Jefferson was enamored of the unknown. (Translation for the diabetic: You need not be enamored—that's a little too much. But you'll do best if you respond to the challenge, look forward to the journey, and see it as an opportunity to learn more about yourself and to live a more, not less, enriched life.)

Since the West was "the wilderness," it held the magic and trepidation the imagination can impart to what we do not know. In other words, he envisioned the West a somewhat different place than it turned out to be. The wisdom of the time had it that as you entered into the wilderness and moved further and further away from "civilization," you also went back in time. There were said to be woolly mammoths in the West and mountains of salt, and Thomas Jefferson believed the rumors and conjectures of the times along with the next American. But that was okay, because his vision of the West and his excitement regarding all that might be found there prompted him to sponsor the Lewis and Clark expedition. He had the intelligence, perspicacity, determination, and drive to want first and foremost to separate reality from rumor and conjecture. (Read this as your disposing of the stereotypes regarding diabetes by investigating the reality of diabetes treatment.)

The journey was hard and took longer than anyone could have imagined. (Remember, this was a 4 mile an hour world. I wonder if that made it less stressful. No, there were probably equally viable stresses—using an outhouse in the middle of the night, for example, or having no outhouse at all.) News of the expedition was slow in getting to the president. Many who knew of the expedition gave up hope, but not Jefferson. He never wavered. (This is a heavy handed message to "keep the faith," or to hew to your program.)

When news did come, it was not at all what he had thought it would be. Instead of the tusk of a woolly mammoth, Lewis and Clark sent him a prairie dog. (At least they spared him the unenchanting gopher.) They also sent back (by slow wagon and slow boat) coyote bones, antelope skeletons, and "Indian" corn. It was a far different West than Jefferson ever imagined. (Read this as no matter how strong the vision or how powerful the person, nobody gets precisely what they want.)

What Lewis and Clark had found was not what Jefferson had bargained for, but it was equally awe inspiring in the end. As the philosopher Heraclitus said, "You must expect the unexpected." In modern terminology, when Jefferson had to switch gears, he did. He was excited by the possibilities and potential of the land, the game, the resources, even though you might say after all the lovely rumors, the truth came at him out of left field, or in this case, the West. (That one's easy. Whatever it is, even if it's diabetes, make the most of it.)

By the time the expedition reached what is now Washington State, many of the men had contracted syphilis, but there were no diary entries of any illnesses that resembled diabetes. (I'll take diabetes.)

When the men returned, they were honored by the president, who was as pleased with the results of the expedition as he would have been if all had turned out as he expected. (You might say, "We may not get what we love, but in the end, we must love what we get.")

We won't talk about what happened to poor Meriweather Lewis, who seems to have irrationally felt himself a failure. He may have benefited from modern antidepressant drugs. He may not have. But it is impossible not to honor him by quoting the most popularized line in the journals of Lewis and Clark, and one that was certainly an unspoken mantra of President Thomas Jefferson's as well: "We proceeded on."

CONSCIOUS LIVING

Managing your diabetes is a daily proposition, a composite of physical acts and disciplined decisions, a practical matter, a health issue you manage with your doctor. But it is more than that. To take control of the situation is also to make a commitment to yourself, your future, your family and friends. And—not to grind the wheel of spirituality too hard—such a commitment to personal discipline can be an invitation to live a more highly conscious and, therefore, fulfilling life. Instead of limiting your horizons, managing your diabetes well can expand them.

You've made a personal journey, albeit an internal one, that has taken you from a starting point of feeling a lack of control over your own health to the destination of knowing you can affect change in your own life and assert control. What you've attained is power, not the power of money or might, but real power that comes from within, from knowing you can do what you have to do. Obviously, such a sense of confidence comes and goes. We're all human, and to be human is to live with fallibility and weaknesses as well as inspiration and strength. There are still days when I beat myself up over every little thing. There are days when I feel I haven't attained even the most rudimentary goals. But these moods don't last as long as they once did, and I do find I choose my battles more carefully and enjoy the little things in life a little bit more. Anyone who has gone through a personal health crisis has the opportunity to experience a newfound appreciation for life. I feel lucky as a diabetic that I can manage my disease and still retain this heightened appreciation of life. Remember, not all diseases respond so generously to the diligent efforts of the patient toward self-care. Of course, it's all in how you see it, but I would say that we're lucky.

Life isn't perfect, and neither is the day-to-day business of managing diabetes. But it's better than the alternative, which is not trying and paying the consequences of out-of-control blood glucose levels and poor health. Take a page from my book. I always fall down on the job. I just never call it failure. This allows me to try again. If I can do this, you can do this, too. Changing our lives happens in increments at best. And you can only change your life if you trust the increments. If you give up because progress is slow, there will be no progress. If you keep going, a little progress will mount up to a lot.

Trust me, I'm not there yet. Probably neither are you. And that's okay. We're on our way. And that's what counts.

I'm not saying diabetes will help you discover the secret of life, but it can give you an edge when it comes to enjoying simple pleasures. I see things differently now. I look at the faces of people who are still suffering the "doom and gloom" of everyday life and living life as an obstacle course, and I can only smile. There is nothing like a crisis in your life to free you from living every day as a perpetual crisis. Whenever I fall into the "I've got a hard life" blues, I remind myself of what I've accomplished close to home, that is, maintaining my health. And I tell myself this is no small thing. This allows me to maintain twenty-twenty vision when it comes to seeing the joy and the pleasure in life.

I won't make too much out of diabetes as a transcendent experience, but I'll say this. You might as well use it as one. It beats the heck out of falling into despair and buying the stereo-type. Sure diabetes can make you sick, but you don't have to let it. Sure the complications can be ugly, but you don't have to get them. Sure diabetes is a disease, but it doesn't have to be a ter-minal one. Your self-determination can make all the difference. You are facing a situation in which control can be yours as long as you take it. Fundamentally, you have a choice; having a choice gives you power. And not every situation in life provides you with a choice. You might say then that diabetes could be seen as an existential dilemma as well as a medical condition. It is your prison, but it is a prison in which you can become free.

When you manage your diabetes well, you should feel exhilarated, and you should be proud of yourself. You've changed the course of your life. You may not have scaled the World Trade Center or broken the sound barrier in a car, but you've done what Candide so wisely advised. You've cultivated your garden—in this case, your health. Now, may all good things grow.

In the twenty-first century, we can all envision a world in which fewer and fewer diabetics suffer the terrible complications of the disease. We may also be able to predict a world in which more and more diabetics can manage their disease with diet and exercise. And most definitely we can predict a world in which preventing diabetes becomes as much of a common cause in America as preventing heart disease and in which a cure for diabetes is not a concept, but a reality. And each one of us is part of that future. As tough as diabetes may be for you, try to imagine how much you can do for future generations of diabetics by doing as well as you can. We are the people who can show to others that diabetes need not be a depressing, terminal disease. We have a choice. And our choice will change how the world views diabetes.

MOTIVATIONAL TIPS

Here are some motivational tips to take you on your journey:

- If you gave up yesterday, don't give up today.
- You save for retirement, right? Well, consider calling this program the healthiest investment you can make in your future. Do a little bit every day and watch your dividends build.
- Many of us take better care of our houses than we do our bodies. Remember your body is your primary home. Take good care of it and living there will be far more pleasant.

- Scarlet O'Hara was right, or never go hungry to a party. Whether or not tomorrow is another day may be debatable, but Scarlet was right about eating before going to the gala ball. Now, had she been a diabetic, she would have been in more trouble than if she had starved herself, since, I believe, she chowed down on about a quart of ice cream. Nevertheless, it makes sense to have a high-protein snack before going to a party, where all manner of tempting morsels may be served that could sway you from your appointed, healthy path.

- Have snack, will travel. Always pack a small plastic bag of almonds in your briefcase or shoulder bag. This can tide you over when you become hungry at inopportune times. (I was in my lawyer's office with my husband and his lawyer and felt queasy with hunger. I went to the restroom, scarfed down my preferred lucky number's worth of nuts, seven, and returned to the meeting a whole lot more stable.) If you are insulin dependent, your snack bag should include a higher carbohydrate food—say a piece of whole grain bread, or a muffin, or bran or wheat crackers. You should work out the ideal "salvation snack" for your insulin regimen with your doctor.

- The race is to the slow. Don't eat anything in a minute that you can eat in half an hour. The slower you eat, the easier the job is for insulin to metabolize the glucose that is coming its way. So, in the case of diabetes, whether yours involves insulin resistance (Type II) or the impairment of beta cells resulting in less insulin (Type I), less is more than more. Sending insulin its work in smaller amounts can help to keep blood glucose levels from rising rapidly.

- Have Glucometer, will travel. Even if your blood glucose levels are humming along at precisely normal, take your

Glucometer wherever and whenever you travel. When you're on vacation, just having your trusty kit with you may help serve to check your desire to cheat on yourself with sweets and other simple carbohydrates that will hit your blood hard.

- Take a vacation day. Spa Diabetes may never be the rage, but taking a day off from work to invest in yourself and your new life-changing regime can help you get off to a good start in managing your diabetes. When you take this "mental health" day, be sure to build rewards into the day for yourself, by which I don't mean eating candy and cookies at breakfast, lunch, and dinner, but rather buying yourself that new tie, or shirt, or CD, or book and taking time for a bubble bath, a round of gold, or a walk in the park.

- Go grocery shopping and take the time (because you have it, you're on vacation right?) to read all the labels.

- Go to a sporting goods store and buy free weights.

- Go to a video store and buy a recommended weight-training video.

- Go to the bookstore and research the diabetes and nutrition section. It's okay; I won't be jealous. If you are insulin dependent, *Dr. Bernstein's Diabetes Solution* can be particularly valuable. *Protein Power*, by Drs. Michael and Mary Dan Eades, is also a great resource and will help to quickly reorient you from carbohydrate overload to a more sensible, protein rich diet.

- Whether you're in the bath or sitting at a cafe with your favorite flavor coffee, read this book.

- Breathe through your stress. If and when you are experiencing a moment of acute stress, you may or may not notice that you have tendency to breathe more shallowly and even to hold your breath for a moment. Whether or not you notice, these phenomena are true. And when we breathe shallowly and less regularly, we take in less oxygen—just when we need it the most.

- When you feel pressured and sense your stress level rising, concentrate specifically on your breathing. Think about inhaling as you do so. Try to focus on the precise moment you then begin to exhale. Think about exhaling. Try to focus on the precise moment you then begin to inhale. Repeat the cycle, inhaling and exhaling, marking the two moments when the cycle of breath changes. As you do so, you will find you begin to breathe more deeply. You'll get more oxygen, and you will be able to shut out the cacophony and babble around you for a moment while you regain your equilibrium. This may or may not help keep your blood glucose levels from raging, but it will certainly aid you in keeping your mental balance and protect you from bouts of panic in which you might feel compelled to go down to the newsstand or corner deli for a treat to relieve your tension—using your stress as an excuse to stress your body further. Breathe instead. Not only is breathing essential, but it has no calories, and there is an art to doing it well. And "inhale-exhale" is a perfect mantra. It has yin-yang written all over it.

- Use cue cards. If you have trouble remembering your no-no's and yes-yes's when you leave home, write down a list on 3-by-5-inch index cards of what goes and what doesn't go. Depending on your personality type, it can be as general or as detailed as you like. For example, a generalist may be able to get by with one card that gives the list of absolute no's, one with the near no's, and one with what goes. The more intense type A may want to correlate foods and portion sizes, percentages, and grams, depending on the desired level of detail. This is one way to avoid ever using the excuse, "Oh, but I forgot."

Index

6 months, 182–184
dietary plan, 161–186
  See also diet diary
  cravings, dealing with,
    168–169
  daily strategy, 163–165
  and family eating, 189–190
  fast starter, 171
  funnel approach, 186
  individual plan, 165–169
  indulgences, 177–178
  medium starter, 171–172
  nutritional percentages,
    165–167, 180, 185
  and other health problems,
    210–211
  physical changes caused by,
    170, 178–179
  portion sizes, 177, 178–179
  precautions, 169
  restrictions, 162, 166–167,
    170–171, 177
  slow starter, 172
  starting tips, 163, 165–166
  and your personality, 170–172
digestion
  and alcoholic beverages, 165,
    196–197
  problems with, 102, 103, 127
digestive enzymes, 132
dining tips, 207–209
dinner parties, and diabetic
  diet, 207–209, 255
dips, 203, 206–207
diuretics, 79
doctor's supervision, importance of, 101
dosage requirements, of insulin,
  33–34
Dr. Bernstein's Diabetes

Solution, xv, 36, 163, 200, 256
drugs, 37
  See also insulin; oral hypo-
    glycemic agents
  antidepressants, 79
  caffeine, 198–199
  prescribed, 78–79
  recreational, 79
  tobacco, 80
dysmenorrhea, 23

E
Eades, Michael R. and Mary
  Dan, 163
ejaculation, retrograde, 75
endocrine system, 5, 8–9, 32
endocrinologist, 135–136
endurance, 24–25
environmental factors, for diabetes, 15
enzymes, digestive, 132
epinephrine, 66, 121
estrogen, 92
exchanges, dietary, 145–146
exercise, 165, 167, 215–216
  adding to daily routine,
    217–221
  aerobic, 228–229, 234–235
  anaerobic, 228–233,
    235–236
  and blood glucose levels,
    223, 223–224
  calories burned during, 237
  and circulation, 116
  cool down and warm up,
    218–219, 222–223
  cross-training, 234
  motivation for, 238–239
  regimen, 176, 233–237
  safety, 222–227

protein, 149–151, 152–153
  amino acids, 150
  calories of, 144
  and diet, 165–166
  and insulin, 150
  requirements, 152–153
  and vegetarians, 151
Protein Power, 163, 200, 256
pulse, taking your, 221

R
recipes, 199–203
reflexology, 133–134, 135
research on diabetes, vii, 42
  amylin, 45–46
  in cloning beta cells, 47
  implantable insulin devices,
    46–47
  insulin therapy, 45
restaurant dining, 178–179, 192
retinopathy, 101, 103–106, 222
retrograde ejaculation, 75
rice, 162
risk factors, 9–10, 14–15, 17
Robinson, Jo, 155
Rose, W. C., 152

S
salads, 201–202
salt, 199
sandwiches, 198–199
saturated fat, 150, 152–153, 155
sedentary lifestyle, 4, 8, 15
self-destructive behaviors,
  68–70, 170–172
sexual function, 71–78
  and aging, 76–78
  and contraception, 75–76
  impotence, 72–75
  and insulin pumps, 78

men's fertility, 75
  and safe sex, 78
shin spots, 110
shrimp salad nicoise, 201
Simopoulos, Artemis P., 155
Sisyphus, 215
skin care, 110–111
smoking, 80
somatostatin, 8
spices, 189
spinning, 228
static activity. *See* anaerobic
  exercise
statistics, on diabetes, 3–4
stereotypes, about diabetes,
  42–45
sterilization, 76
stress, 15–16, 23
  and adrenaline, 66–67
  and blood glucose levels,
    65–67
  and dealing with crisis, 68
  and the immune system, 66
  and massage, 135
  and overall health, 67
  reducers, 67, 256–257
stretching exercises, 218–219
strokes, 101, 106
support groups, 28–29
surgery, 137
sweeteners, artificial, 162, 167,
  208
sweets, 202–203, 208–209
symptoms, of diabetes, 12

T
teeth, caring for your, 117–119
thirst, excessive, 12
"tight control", 41, 100,
  245–246